INTERMITTENT
FASTING BIBLE
for Women over 50

The complete guide to boost your metabolism, lose weight and improve your eating habits with healthy and clean meals.

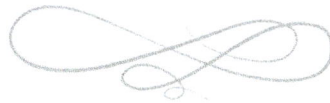

MARY LIGHT

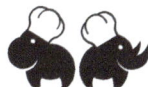

IPPOCERONTE
publishing

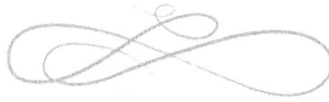

Contents

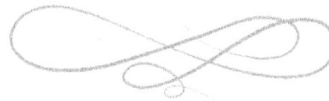

Introduction

Intermittent fasting has several advantages that make it ideal for women as they age. Not only do women struggle to lose weight as their metabolism slows as they age, but they are also more susceptible to a variety of age- and weight-related ailments. We'll go over some of the best reasons to choose this lifestyle in detail. This will allow you to determine if it is a good fit for you.

The first advantage of intermittent fasting is that it helps you feel full while eating less food. Studies show that intermittent fasting helps to shed pounds and reduce belly fat in roughly equal measure. By avoiding the constant need to eat, this diet minimizes the chances of overeating or feeling dissatisfied with your food. Forcing yourself to eat smaller portions, especially at breakfast when your appetite tends to be the strongest, is a surefire way to lose weight.

WEIGHT LOSS

While many people attempt diet after diet in the hopes of losing weight, they are more likely to succeed with intermittent fasting. After all, while the human body is normally forced to burn off the food we have eaten on a regular basis, when you are fasted, you can work on burning off your body fat instead.

METABOLIC RESET

Many women, as they age, experience reduced metabolism. The best way to correct this is by resetting your metabolism, which is exactly what intermittent fasting does. For those unfamiliar with the concept of metabolism, it is the way that your body uses food for energy. Intermittent fasting allows you to reduce both of these actions, so you have less stored body fat and more usable energy from food.

Intermittent fasting has several advantages that make it ideal for women as they age. Not only do women struggle to lose weight as their metabolism slows as they age, but they are also more susceptible to a variety of age- and weight-related ailments. We'll go over some of the best reasons to choose this lifestyle in detail. This will allow you to determine if it is a good fit for you.

The first advantage of intermittent fasting is that it helps you feel full while eating less food. Studies show that intermittent fasting helps to shed pounds and reduce belly fat in roughly equal measure. By avoiding the constant need to eat, this diet minimizes the chances of overeating or feeling dissatisfied with your food. Forcing yourself to eat smaller portions, especially at breakfast when your appetite tends to be the strongest, is a surefire way to lose weight.

WEIGHT LOSS

While many people attempt diet after diet in the hopes of losing weight, they are more likely to succeed with intermittent fasting. After all, while the human body is normally forced to burn off the food we have eaten on a regular basis, when you are fasted, you can work on burning off your body fat instead.

METABOLIC RESET

Many women, as they age, experience reduced metabolism. The best way to correct this is by resetting your metabolism, which is exactly what intermittent fasting does. For those unfamiliar with the concept of metabolism, it is the way that your body uses food for energy. Intermittent fasting allows you to reduce both of these actions, so you have less stored body fat and more usable energy from food.

INCREASE HUMAN GROWTH HORMONE

HGH, or Human Growth Hormone, is a hormone that many people lose as they get older. Although many other hormones decline as you get older, this is one that you can actively improve by making small lifestyle changes. During your fast, you will take extra doses of this hormone to help repair your worn and damaged tissues.

CONVERT YOUR BODY FAT

When you fast, your body is able to burn body fat much more effectively than when you eat. This is due to the fact that most of our body's cells are unable to use glucose as a primary energy source because they are often working while you sleep and lack the energy to exercise. Intermittent fasting allows your cells to use fat for fuel, which results in weight loss.

IMPROVE MUSCLE HEALTH

When you are fasting, your body does not have the resources to work out as many times per week as it would if you were eating. While your muscles do not rely on glucose for energy, they do rely on protein for a greater portion of their requirements. Fasting allows your body to more effectively use stored protein to produce the energy required by your muscles, making them stronger and healthier.

BOOSTED ENERGY
You may find that when you fast, your energy levels are much higher than when you eat. The reason for this is that fasting burns glucose out of your system, preventing it from being used as a source of energy. When you're hungry, you'll be compelled to look for food rather than take on the task of burning off the sugar in your body. This leads to more coherent and optimal energy levels throughout the day, as well as a healthier lifestyle overall.

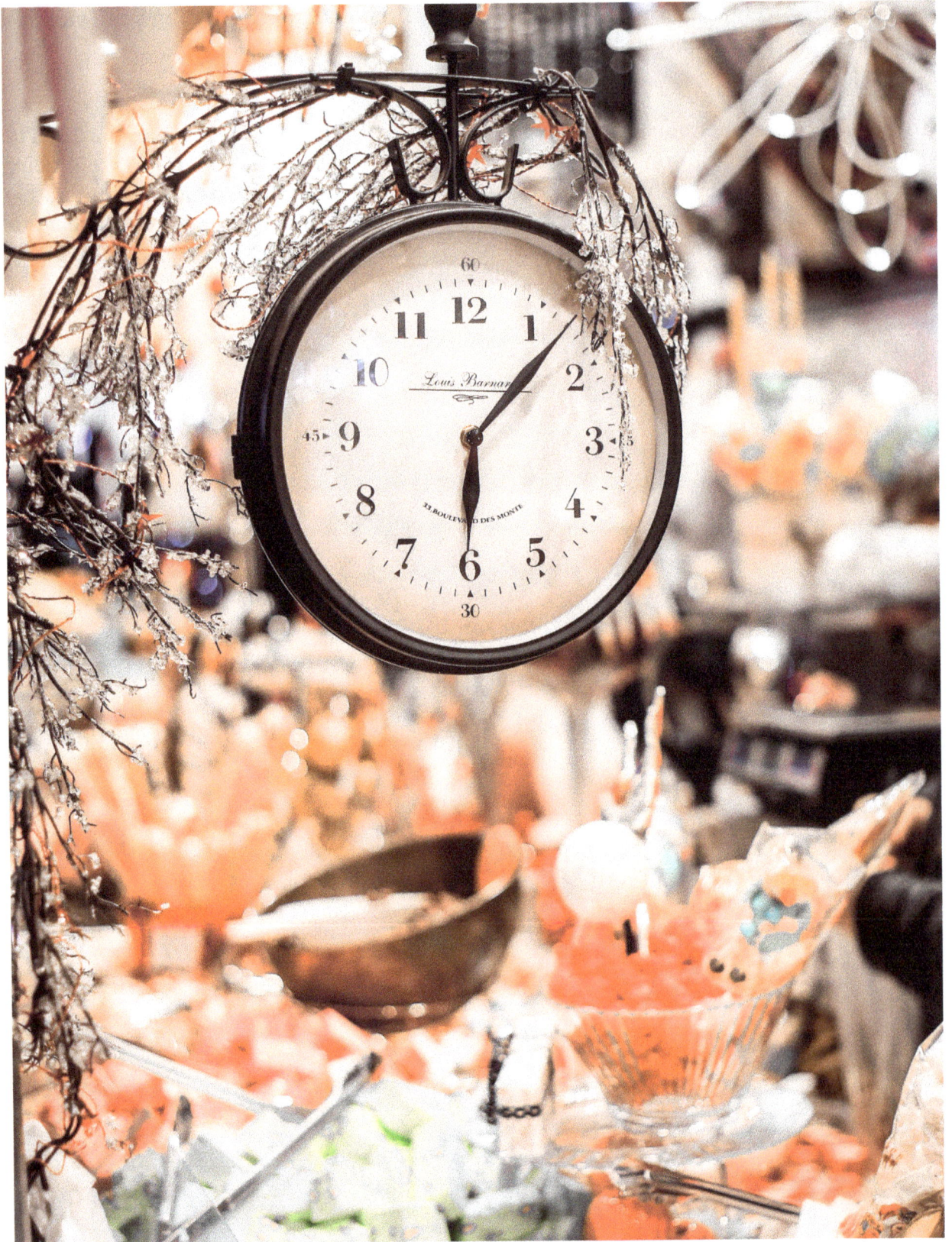

CHAPTER I

Intermittent Fasting for Women Over 50

It's becoming increasingly harder for a woman to lose weight after the age of 50, and we're obsessed with those extra pounds that pile up in places we don't want them to, such as hips and love handles. Intermittent fasting is a diet that differs from traditional diets. When you consider the numerous health and mental benefits of calorie restriction, it can also become a way of life. The various intermittent fasting types allow us to assess and select the best one for us, tailoring it to our specific needs and lifestyle.

To begin this type of "diet," you must first be in good health, and it is always best to consult your doctor before beginning. Because the hypothalamus, a brain gland responsible for hormone production, is stimulated, the female body is vulnerable to calorie limitation. With a dramatic reduction in calories or a fast that lasts too long, these hormones may go haywire.

HOW INTERMITTENT FASTING AFFECTS YOUR WEIGHT

Intermittent fasting not only affects your metabolism, but it can also aid weight loss. When you go without food for a long time, your body starts to burn more fat and less muscle. You'll begin to lose weight as your body begins to remove fat from your own tissues in order to conserve energy for other functions. Fasting causes your body to burn more of its own tissue in order to sustain normal processes and functions.

WHAT IS INTERMITTENT FASTING

Intermittent fasting is a way to lose weight by consuming calories during a short period of time. The daily intake is severely restricted, and the 24-hour fast is interrupted by periods of eating. Some people only eat from 12 noon until 8 p.m., which is called the "lean gains method" after the fitness website on which it's promoted, while others stop eating after 6 p.m.—which is generally known as "16:8".

How does IF work

Intermittent fasting has been around for a long time, and different variants of the method have emerged over time. It works by balancing you're eating window with periods of fasting to regulate your blood sugar levels.

After completing a fast, most people report feeling more energized, allowing them to increase their physical activity. You'll have better insulin sensitivity and blood sugar control after doing intermittent fasting. Insulin is released in response to a variety of foods, especially carbohydrates.

Intermittent Fasting and its Effect on Metabolism

Fasting for short periods of time is believed to help your metabolism.
It does not speed up your metabolism; rather, it increases the efficiency with which you burn calories. The body is forced to adjust to extreme calorie restriction during an intermittent fasting session.

In order to survive, it must regulate its calorie-burning by reducing hunger and increasing the breakdown of fat reserves. When you place food in front of your body, it will attempt to break it down and utilize its energy first.

What Happens to Women's Bodies After 50?

After the age of 50, our bodies slow down. Our cells start to become less sensitive to insulin, which means that our bodies cannot regulate blood sugar levels as well as they used to. The process of burning stored fat and muscle for energy is slower than it was in our teens and twenties.

Keeping this in mind, there have been several studies carried out examining what intermittent fasting does for women over the age of 50. In one study, it was discovered that women aged over 50 who regularly fasted for 16 hours a day lost over 3 pounds in their first week of following the diet plan.

Menopause and Intermittent Fasting

As a woman reaches her forties and fifties, she goes menopause, her hormones gradually decrease as her ovaries stop producing estrogen and progesterone, preventing menstruation. She is said to have entered menopause because she hasn't had a cycle for 12 months, but amenorrhea isn't the only symptom of menopause.

After menopause, women may become less receptive to insulin, as if the other signs weren't enough, and they may have difficulty absorbing sugar and processed carbohydrates; this physiologic transition is known as insulin resistance, and it is associated with fatigue and sleep difficulties.

Fortunately, women may use intermittent fasting as a method to help them handle the slowing roller coast of menopause. During the menopause journey, you might want to give it a try if you're dealing with exhaustion, weight gain, or insulin resistance.

BENEFITS AND RISK OF INTERMITTENT FASTING FOR WOMEN OVER 50

It has been proven that intermittent fasting aids in weight loss. Fasting increases insulin sensitivity and makes the body absorb sugar and carbohydrates more efficiently, lowering the risk of heart disease, diabetes, and other metabolic diseases

Benefits of Intermittent fasting for women over 50
- It helps fix cellular forms in your body.
- It advances weight reduction, particularly gut fat.
- It helps lessens aggravation and oxidative pressure.
- It may help forestall Alzheimer's infection.
- It may broaden your life

Potential Risk of Intermittent fasting for women over 50
- Extreme Hunger
- No Focus on Nutritious Eating
- May Promote Overeating
- Long haul Limitations

Intermittent fasting can have serious consequences if people fast when they shouldn't. Intermittent fasting, on the other hand, isn't very dangerous for most people. You'll be at risk of bingeing, malnutrition, and trouble keeping the fast going.

Malnutrition may sound frightening, but you can avoid it for the most part by eating well-balanced meals during your eating windows. Malnutrition is a risk, particularly during fasting days with a very low-calorie restriction.

Dehydration is linked to malnutrition. The food we eat provides a significant portion of our daily water intake. However, if you're eating less food or no meal during the day, you'll need to drink a lot more water than usual.

One of the dangers associated with fasting is that it can be difficult to get started. During the first few weeks of following your fasting schedule, you will be hungry. Mood swings, irregular bowel movements, and sleep disturbances may make you feel uneasy. These emotions should not be dismissed at the outset. If you are experiencing extreme discomfort while fasting, you should stop and consult your doctor.

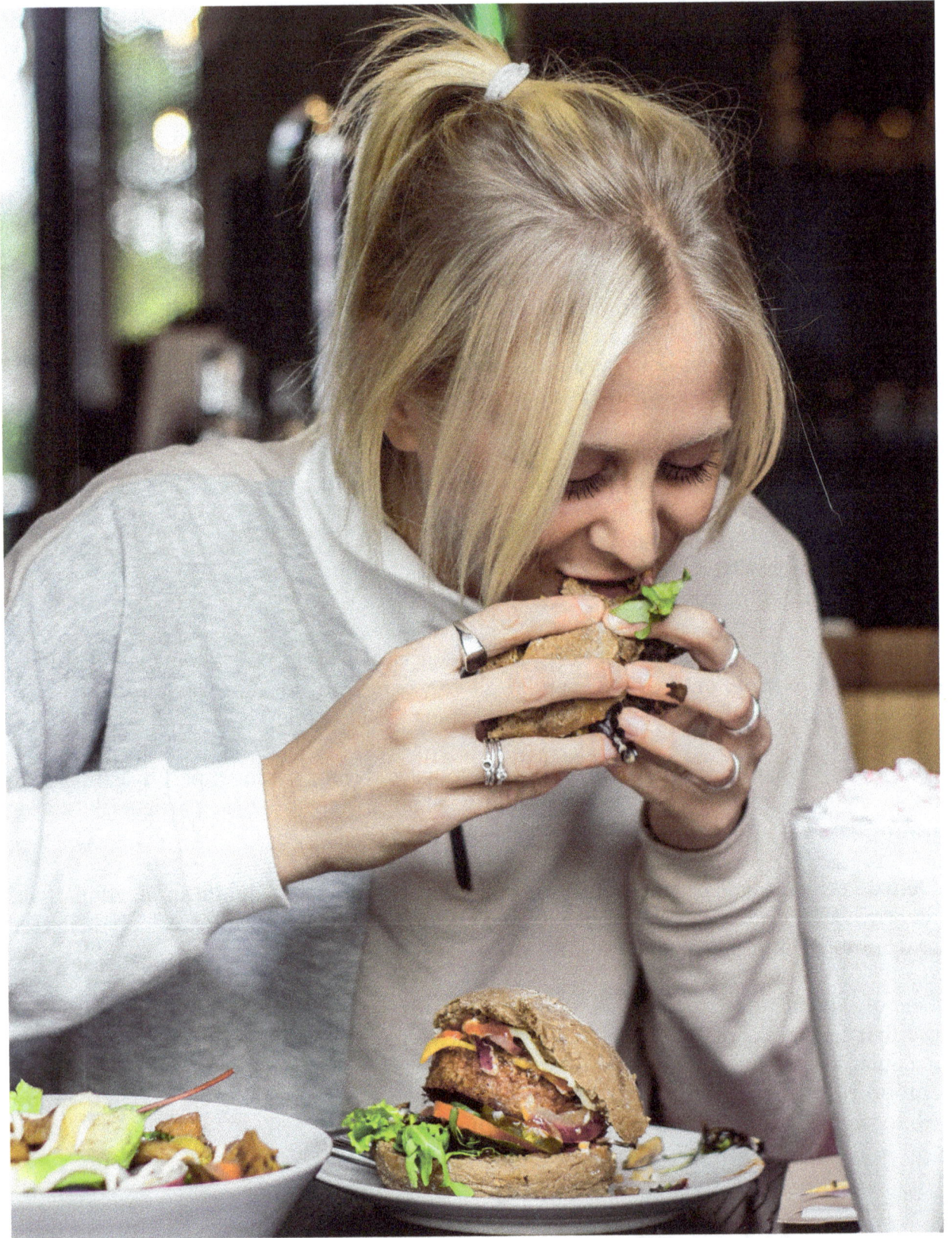

CHAPTER 2

The right type of intermittent fasting

16/8 METHOD

This is just about the most popular fasting methods since it's so schedule based, meaning there are no surprises. This will give you the freedom to control when you eat based on the everyday life of yours. The sixteen is the number of hours you're likely to be fasting, which may also be lowered to twelve or perhaps fourteen hours if that fits into your life better. Then your eating period is going to be between eight and ten hours every day. This might seem daunting, but it just means that you are skipping an entire meal. Many people choose to begin their fast around 7 or 8 p.m. and then do not eat until 11 or noon the next day, which means they fast for the recommended 16 hours. Of course, it isn't as bad as it sounds since they are sleeping during this time, so what it comes down to is eating dinner and then not eating the next day again around lunch, so you are just skipping breakfast.

You will be doing it every day, so finding the hours that work for you are important. If you work the third shift, then switching your eating period around to fit into your schedule is important. If you find yourself being run down and sluggish, tweak your fasting hours until you find a healthy balance. Granted, there will be some adjustment because chances are, your body is not accustomed to skipping entire meals. However, this should go away after a couple of weeks, and if it doesn't, then try starting your fasting period earlier in the day, allowing you to eat earlier the next, or alter it however you need to feel healthy and happy.

LEAN-GAINS METHOD (14:10)

The lean-gains method has several different incarnations on the web, but its fame comes from the fact that it helps shed fat while building it into muscle almost immediately. Through the lean-gains method, you'll find yourself able to shift all that fat to be muscle through a rigorous practice of fasting, eating right, and exercising.

Through this method, you fast anywhere from 14 to 16 hours and spend the remaining 10 or 8 hours each day engaged in eating and exercise. As opposed to the crescendo, this method features daily fasting and eating, rather than alternated days of eating versus not. Therefore, you don't have to be quite cautious about extending the physical effort to exercise on the days you are fasting because those days when you're fasting are every day!

For the lean-gaining method, start fasting only for 14 hours and work it up to 16 if you feel comfortable with it, but never forget to drink enough water and be careful about spending too much energy on exercise! Remember that you want to grow in health and potential through intermittent fasting. You'll certainly not want to lose any of that growth by forcing the process along.

20:4 METHOD
Stepping things up a notch from the 14:10 and 16:8 methods, the 20:4 method is a tough one to master, for it is rather unforgiving. People talk about this method of intermittent fasting as intense and highly restrictive. Still, they also say that the effects of living this method are almost unparalleled with all other tactics.

For the 20:4 method, you'll fast for 20 hours each day and squeeze all your meals, all your eating, and all your snacking into 4 hours. People who attempt 20:4 normally have two smaller meals or just one large meal and a few snacks during their 4-hour window to eat, and it is up to the individual which four hours of the day they devote to eating.

The trick for this method is to make sure you're not overeating or bingeing during those 4-hour windows to eat. It is all-too-easy to get hungry during the 20-hour fast and have that feeling then propel you into intense and unrealistic hunger or meal sizes after the fast period is over. Be careful if you try this method. If you're new to intermittent fasting, work your way up to this one gradually, and if you're working your way up already, only make the shift to 20:4 when you know you're ready. It would surely disappoint if all your progress with intermittent fasting got hijacked by one poorly thought-out goal with the 20:4 method.

MEAL SKIPPING
Meal skipping is an extremely flexible form of intermittent fasting that can provide all of the benefits of intermittent fasting but with less strict scheduling. If you are not someone who has a typical schedule or feels like a stricter variation of the intermittent fasting diet will serve you, meal skipping is a viable alternative.

Many people who choose to use meal skipping find it a great way to listen to their bodies and follow their basic instincts. If they are not hungry, they simply don't eat that meal. Instead, they wait for the next one. Meal skipping can also help people who have time constraints and who may not always be able to get in a certain meal of the day.

It is important to realize that with meal skipping, you may not always be maintaining a 10-16-hour window of fasting. As a result, you may not get every benefit that comes from other fasting diets. However, this may be a great solution for people who want an intermittent fasting diet that feels more natural. It may also be a great idea for those looking to begin listening to their bodies more so that they can adjust to a more extreme variant of the diet with greater ease. It can be a great transitional diet for you if you are not ready to jump into one of the other fasting diets just yet.

WARRIOR DIET FASTING

The most extreme form of intermittent fasting is known as the Warrior Diet. This intermittent fasting cycle follows a 20-hour fasting window with a short 4-hour eating window. During that eating window, individuals are supposed only to consume raw fruits and vegetables. They can also eat one large meal. Typically, the eating window occurs at nighttime, so people can snack throughout the evening, have a large meal, and then resume fasting.

Because of the length of fasting taking place during the Warrior Diet, people should also consume a fairly hearty level of healthy fats. Doing so will give the body something to consume during the fast to produce energy with. Additional carbohydrates are also used to increase energy levels; too.

People who eat the Warrior Diet tend to believe that humans are natural nocturnal eaters and that we are not meant to eat throughout the day. The belief is that eating this way follows our natural circadian rhythms, allowing our body to work optimally.

The only people who should consider doing the Warrior Diet are those who have already had success with other forms of intermittent fasting and who are used to it. Attempting to jump straight into the Warrior Diet can have serious repercussions for anyone who is not used to intermittent fasting. Even still, those who are used to it may find this particular style too extreme for them to maintain.

EAT-STOP-EAT (24 HOUR) METHOD

This method of fasting is incredibly similar to the crescendo method. The only discernible difference is that there's no anticipation of increasing into a more intense fasting pattern with time. For the eat-stop-eat method, you decide which days you want to take off from eating, and then you run with it until you've lost that weight, and then you keep running with the lifestyle for good because you won't be able to imagine life without it.

The eat-stop-eat method involves one to two days a week being 100% oriented towards fasting, with the other five to six days concerning "business as normal." The one or two days spent fasting are then full 24-hour days spent without eating anything at all. These days, of course, water and coffee are still fine to drink, but no food items can be consumed whatsoever. Exercise is also frowned upon on those fasting days but see what your body can handle before you decide how that should all work out.

Some people might start thinking they're using the crescendo method but end up sticking with eat-stop-eat.

ALTERNATE-DAY METHOD

The alternate-day method is admittedly a little confusing, but the reason it could be so confusing could come, in part, from how much wiggle room it provides for the practitioner. This method is great for people who don't have a consistent schedule or any sense of one; it is incredibly forgiving for those who don't quite have everything together for themselves yet.

When it comes down to it, alternate-day intermittent fasting is really up to you. You should try to fast every other day, but it doesn't have to be that precise. Similarly, with the crescendo method, as long as you fast two to three days a week, with a break day or two in between each fasting day, you're set! Then, you'll want to eat normally for three or four days out of each week, and when you encounter a fasting day, you don't even need to completely fast!

Alternate-day fasting is a solid place to start from, especially if you work a varying schedule or still have yet to get used to a consistent one. If you want to make things more intense from this starting point, the alternate-day method can easily become the eat-stop-eat method, the crescendo method, or the 5:2 method. Essentially, this method is a great place to begin

12:12 METHOD

As another of the more natural ways of intermittent fasting, the 12:12 approach is well-suited to beginning practitioners. Many people live out the 12:12 method without any forethought simply because of their sleeping and eating schedule but turning 12:12 into a conscious practice can have just as many positive effects on your life as the more drastic 20:4 method claims.

According to a study conducted in the University of Alabama, for this method, in particular, you fast for 12 hours and then enter a 12-hour eating window. It's not difficult whatsoever to get three small meals and several snacks, or two big meals and a snack into your day with this method. With 12:12, the standard meal timing works just fine.

Ultimately, this method is a great one to start from, for a lot of variation can be built into this scheduling when you're ready to make things more interesting. Effortlessly and without much effort, 12:12 can become 14:10 or even 16:8, and in seemingly no time, you can find yourself trying alternate-day or crescendo methods, too. Start with what's normal for you, and this method might be exactly that!

CHAPTER 3

Let's begin

How Do You Start Your Intermittent Fasting?

If you've ever tried to go to the gym or tried dieting, you're probably aware of the bulking and cutting cycles. Well, now it's time to put those in the past and get acquainted with Intermittent Fasting. This is a process that will help you lose weight while gaining muscle. Anyone who has tried Intermittent Fasting agrees that it is an excellent way to lose weight in a manner that doesn't cause us any hunger pangs, distress or health complications like other dieting can cause. Here are the steps to help you begin your Intermittent Fasting Journey:

Create a Monthly Calendar

The first step to determine when you should eat and when you should not be making a calendar for the entire month. This is one way of mapping out your schedule so that you can plan well in advance. The best time to do this is on the first day of the month.

Choose the Right Days

In order to get started, you will need to choose the right days that will work with your schedule. This means that you will need to choose days that are suitable for your schedule.

Record Your Findings

Make sure that you not only jot down the days where you can fast and when you cannot fast but also note all the types of food that should be taken on different days. This is one way of recording your findings so that you can follow through with it.

Follow the Plan

One of the most valuable things when it comes to Intermittent Fasting is to follow the plan. This means that you need to make sure that you devote time for this or else this will turn out as a failed attempt.

Keep A Journal

One of the most valuable things to do when you are Intermittent fasting is writing down all your feelings and emotions. This will help you stay on track. Some people even write down their meals in a journal so that they can keep track of it. This not only helps them remember what they ate but also prevents them from going off the rails and indulging in more food.

Reward Yourself

Since you are now aware of how great this Intermittent Fasting is as a weight loss tool, you will need to reward yourself for working hard. This of course means that you will have to eat something on those days when you do not fast.

Remember, Intermittent fasting works because it is all about timing you're eating and drinking. Fasting for 20 hours per day is perhaps the best way of losing weight without suffering hunger pangs and also developing muscles effectively.

Curb Hunger Pains

One of the best ways to curb hunger pangs is by drinking water. By drinking water, you will be filling your stomach up so that the hunger pangs or cravings are taken care of.

Stay Hydrated

Keeping hydrated is the most important aspect of intermittent fasting. This means that you need to drink water regularly throughout the day. The rule is simple: drink at least thirteen cups of water per day for optimum health and weight loss results.

Stay Busy

One of the most effective ways to keep from getting hungry is by staying busy. This means that you need to keep yourself occupied and prevent yourself from getting bored.

Meet with People

One of the best tools that are available to you when it comes to Intermittent Fasting is talking with people who are also doing this. One way of working through problems or trying to lose weight by eating healthy food would be talking about your success with others who have done it before you.

Practice Mindful Eating

Eating mindfully is one of the most effective ways to combat hunger pangs. This means that you need to be aware of your eating habits and not feel guilty about what you are eating.

Practice Portion Control

One of the most important things that you need to do when it comes to Intermittent Fasting is to be consistent with your portion control. This means that you need to learn how much food is considered a normal serving size and stick with that number.

Get Tech Savvy

While Intermittent Fasting might seem like a simple process, it is very important to get tech savvy. This means that you need to make use of apps and other equipment to help you keep track of what you are eating and when.

Know What to Eat

When it comes to Intermittent Fasting, one of the most important things that you need to do is to know what type of food you should eat when you are fasting.

WRITING DOWN YOUR GOALS

One of the most important things to do when Intermittent fasting and trying to lose weight is to write down all of your goals. This includes how much weight you want to lose, how many days a week you can fast, and what level of activity will help you achieve your goals. People have a common misconception about intermittent fasting in that they believe they can eat whatever they want as long as they fast for the necessary hours every day. This, however, is not the case. While Intermittent Fasting allows you to eat whatever you want, it also requires you to fast for a specified number of hours each day. This means that, after a certain period of time, your body will begin to adapt to the lack of food and, as a result, will become healthier in the long run. It also aids in the fight against cancer cells and the development of certain diseases in your body.

CHOOSING THE RIGHT TYPE OF INTERMITTENT FASTING

Now that you're aware of the different methods of intermittent fasting available to you, it's time to pick one. There are a few things to consider when selecting a method for yourself.

When deciding on an intermittent fasting schedule for yourself, you should ask yourself some questions. I'll walk you through the questions you should ask yourself to decide which intermittent fasting method is best for you.

What is my current daily routine like?

Examine your daily and weekly schedules. This will give you insight into your busiest times of the day and when you will need the most energy.

When am I currently fasting?

While they sleep, everyone is fasting. Do you usually wait until lunch to eat when you wake up? Do you have a small meal but eat early in the morning? A fast, or even a mini fast, is defined as a period of time without eating. Choose these times to incorporate a fasting schedule that will not cause too much disruption to your current lifestyle.

When will I be unable to fast?

The word "afford" is used in this point in an energetic sense. Keep in mind any special obligations that require your energy, such as an after-dinner sports club or early morning meetings, when deciding on a technique. If you have evening obligations that require physical exertion, you probably won't want to skip dinner; however, if you have morning meetings, eating breakfast first might be just what you need to get started.

If you are a person that has both of these, then maybe you will need to fast for 24 hours on the weekend when you have a less demanding schedule, as you need all the energy that food gives you throughout the week.

Is it possible for me to fast for 24 hours?
Without prior experience or an entire day set aside to relax while fasting, not everyone can fast for 24 hours. Are you willing to put in the effort and time required by a 24-hour fast, as well as deal with the potential side effects of lethargy, irritability, headaches, and other symptoms? If that's the case, this method could work for you. If not, it's best to move on to another option.

What are the demands in my life that might be a source of difficulty?
Having children to look after and cook for can make intermittent fasting more difficult. An exercise or sports regimen, a slew of social events, or a lack of time to properly prepare a meal plan may all contribute to weight gain.

Take into account all of these obstacles so that you are prepared to face them all. Prepare ahead of time so that nothing comes as a surprise, and you'll be able to stay on track even when these obstacles arise.

You'll have a better idea of what intermittent fasting plan would work best for you after you've answered all of the above questions. The one that best suits your current way of life will be the least likely to stick and produce positive results.

Remember that the first option you choose does not have to be the one you stick with indefinitely. You can still change the hours, days, or even try a different one if it doesn't work for you for some reason. Autophagy and the positive results you seek will occur as long as you follow an intermittent fasting schedule.

WHEN WILL INTERMITTENT FASTING TAKE EFFECT?
Don't be in a rush, intermittent fasting usually starts to pick up at around six weeks. Remember, it took time to gain weight and, unfortunately, there is no magic pill or supplement that will make it disappear overnight. In the beginning, you will lose inches with intermittent fasting because your body is losing water weight and not actual fat. As stated earlier, you will have to give this a six-week trial before giving up on the diet plan if it doesn't work for you.

KNOW YOUR BMI AND HOW TO CALCULATE IT
Before starting any diet plan, you should know your BMI. This is a measurement of your

weight in comparison to your height that determines whether or not you are overweight. Use an online calculator to figure out if you are in this category accurately. If so, Intermittent Fasting will help drop the unhealthy pounds and reduce your BMI.

To determine your BMI, multiply your weight (lbs.) by 703 and divide by your height (in inches) (in).

After you've computed your BMI, compare it to the body mass index chart to see which category you fall into.

Class	Your BMI Score
Underweight	less than 18.5 points
Normal weight	18.5 – 24.9 points
Overweight	25 – 29.9 points
Class 1 - Obesity	30 – 34.9 points
Class 2 — Obesity	35 – 39.9 points
Class 3 — Extreme obesity	40 + points

MACROS AND HOW TO TRACK THEM

Macros are the foundation of Intermittent Fasting and the means by which you can shed pounds. It will be difficult for you to use Intermittent Fasting effectively and achieve your goals if you do not know how to track your macros. This is a very easy technique to use in order to keep track of your macros correctly.

What exactly are macros? Macros are three basic nutrients that your body requires on a daily basis: carbohydrates, proteins, and fats. These are the foods that will aid in weight loss.

What method do I use to keep track of my macros? A piece of paper and a calculator are required, and you can keep a running log throughout the day to stay on track with your diet. This is an important aspect of intermittent fasting because it helps you to see how many calories you might have left over so that your body can burn fat without losing muscle. Follow these steps to keep track of your macros:

1. Take accurate measurements of your meals. A digital scale is the best tool to use because it can give you an accurate count of your food intake. You can also use a kitchen scale, but keep in mind that kitchen scales are notorious for introducing minor inconsistencies and mistakes during counts.

2. Make a calorie count. This is the most important step in monitoring your macros;

if you don't do it, you won't be able to lose weight or keep the weight off if the plan doesn't work for you.

3. Determine your protein and fat consumption. This is an important step. Intermittent Fasting will not work for you unless you have these two nutrients, and you risk losing muscle and fat mass at the same time. Your macros should be included in the weekly or daily log that you keep of your food intake if you decide to use a food tracker.

4. Calculate your total for the week. This will provide a precise count of your macros. Use trial and error to compare your macros to the ones used in this week's food log if you don't think the product you're using can count correctly.

5. Add up your totals for the day. This is also crucial because it will give you a good idea of how many calories you should be eating in order to lose weight or maintain your current weight loss.

6. Keep track of your calories and macronutrients. Make sure you use the same food product tracker every day so you know exactly what you're eating and burning during the day.

7. Keep track of how much weight you've lost in pounds. To keep track of your weight loss, you should use a scale or just look in the mirror.

8. Increase your workout routine if you're attempting to gain muscle or burn fat while also losing weight.

9. Keep a journal. It's best to keep track of your daily food intake and the number of calories you consume because this will be difficult to maintain in the long run if you don't.

BREAKING YOUR FAST

Because all of the fasts in this book are sporadic and not long-term, you can pretty much do whatever you want to break your fast. Nonetheless, there are some factors to consider when determining how to break your fast so that the benefits continue to flow.

Choose foods that are high in nutrients. Plan out how you'll prepare or obtain a nutrient-dense meal that fits your diet plan. If you're out and about or just really hungry when you're breaking your fast, for example, you may want to eat a small snack until you can eat your scheduled meal. Healthy smoothies or soups, such as the Green Smoothie with Apple, Avocado, and Spinach or Spicy Cauliflower Soup, are excellent choices because they are high in nutrients and fiber. They will also help you avoid overeating by filling your stomach. A tablespoon of coconut oil, MCT oil, or another healthy fat is another choice. Maintain your diet. If you're on a ketogenic diet, for example, choose a meal that fits your macros.
Avoid empty calories, refined carbohydrates, and ultra-processed foods, as they will not provide your body with the nourishing nutrients it requires after a fast. If you want your body

to rebuild stronger during the growing phase, avoid foods that provide damaged building blocks, such as trans fats and inflammation-inducing vegetable oils. Cakes, cookies, white bread, pasta, pies, processed foods, sugary drinks, diet sodas, vegetable oil sources, and margarine should all be replaced with real whole foods and natural drinks that fit your diet.

Avoid consuming alcoholic beverages. When breaking a fast, it's not a good idea to drink booze. If you choose to drink alcohol before your first meal, keep in mind that it will intensify the effects, so wait until after you've eaten or paired it with food.

WHAT TO DRINK: PRACTICING INTERMITTENT FASTING FOR WEIGHT LOSS

1. Tea
If you enjoy tea, you'll be pleased to learn that this hot beverage goes hand in hand with the goal of intermittent fasting. Here are some of the advantages:

It aids in the reduction of hunger.

It's a colossal point! We are hungry because we do not eat as much as we should. This is due to an imbalance of the hunger hormone, ghrelin. If we want to feel less hungry, we must return to this balance.

2. Coffee
This contains caffeine, which boosts alertness and aids in weight loss. Caffeine, on the other hand, increases metabolism and aids weight loss.

As a result, drinking coffee while fasting is a great way to control hunger and burn more fat.

3. Apple Cider Vinegar
Most apple cider vinegar is made up of water and acids like acetic acid and malic acid. Appropriately 3 calories are contained in 15 ml (one tablespoon) of apple cider vinegar. Ideal for weight loss!

WHAT TO DRINK: AUTOPHAGY REQUIRES INTERMITTENT FASTING.
Autophagy is a human body process that involves the disposal of old, damaged cells. If these cells remain in the body, they cause inflammation, which can lead to other health problems.

The intermittent fasting helps to clean the body by stimulating autophagy.

Green tea contains active phenols such as epigallocatechin gallate (EGCG) and caffeine, all of which work together to give you an extra boost of energy!

Bone Broth - Combining bone broth consumption with intermittent fasting results in glowing skin, improved hair and nails, reduced inflammation, and a slowed aging process.

Whether you desire to shed some pounds or increase your overall health, bone broth is a must-have in your diet.

EXERCISING WHILE FASTING

While exercising while intermittent fasting can be challenging, there are ways to make it easier. Women over 50 should consider combining exercise and intermittent fasting. What's the best way to combine exercise and intermittent fasting for women over 50?

The key is to avoid overeating after a workout. It is not necessary to eat right after you finish exercising; instead, wait at least a couple of hours and then eat a small, light meal. For example, if you worked out in the morning, save your meal for around noon or later and include some protein and vegetables.

The advantages of combining intermittent fasting with exercise can be significant. Intermittent fasting aids weight loss by increasing fat burning. If you combine exercise with intermittent fasting on a regular basis, you'll be able to lose weight faster because your metabolism will stay elevated and you'll burn even more calories. Many women have reported losing several pounds in a short period of time by combining intermittent fasting with regular exercise.

Intermittent fasting has the advantage of not jeopardizing your workout routine, as some fad diets do. When you fast, you don't get the negative side effects that other fad diets do, which can make it difficult to stick to your workout routine. You can eat whatever you want and not worry about it interfering with your workouts if you use intermittent fasting.

Cardio

There are many benefits of doing cardio exercise, but for women over 50 years old there are also some specific benefits associated with cardio exercise. Cardio exercise helps reduce the risk of heart disease and stroke. When women over 50 years old do cardio exercise, it keeps their cardiovascular system strong, which will help prevent heart disease and stroke. Women over 50 years old who have a healthy lifestyle can play an important role in the prevention of heart disease and stroke.

Cardio exercise 1: JUMPING

When you jump with your entire body, your muscles work harder because they have become used to the stress, resulting in a faster metabolism. Your muscles will become stronger and more toned as you move your body more during the day, such as by running or walking. You should work up to 30 minutes of cardio exercise many times per week.

Cardio exercise 2: RUNNING/JOGGING

Running or jogging is one of the best cardio exercises for women over 50 who do not participate in other forms of exercise. Running or jogging may not be appropriate for younger women in their 20s and 30s, but it is a wonderful way to keep your body fit and healthy if you are over 50. During the run, you will burn more calories, giving you more energy throughout the day. You should increase the amount of time you run based on the amount of time you have available due to your work schedule or other obligations.

Weight Training

Women over the age of 50 will also benefit from weight training's improved bone wellbeing. It also aids in the growth of lean muscle tissue. You will burn lots of calories during the day as a result of this.

Weightlifting helps you build and repair muscles, which is essential for maintaining a healthy body in your fifties. Weight training will assist you in maintaining a healthy weight and enhancing your metabolism. Strength training should be done once or twice a week for 30 to 45 minutes.

Exercises that you can do at home

Women who don't have time to go to the gym can still lose weight by doing a variety of exercises at home.

1. Yoga

Yoga is a good exercise for women over 50 because it improves flexibility. Yoga can assist you in a variety of ways, including improving your sleep. If you're looking for a way to boost your energy throughout the day, try doing yoga first thing in the morning instead of doing cardio. When done too soon after breakfast, some aerobic exercises can actually be counterproductive.

2. Calisthenics

Calisthenics is a great way for women over 50 to lose weight quickly. Push-ups, pull-ups, sit-ups, and squats are examples of exercises that can be done without any equipment. Calisthenics is a simple at-home workout that will help you lose weight quickly. The beauty of calisthenics is that they don't take up a lot of time. Calisthenics may be done in the morning, evening, or even at night before bed.

3. Dance

Dancing is also a good choice for women over 50 who don't have a lot of time because it burns calories while still being enjoyable. Dancing should refer to any kind of dance you enjoy doing, not just ballroom dancing. It can aid in balance, flexibility, and incorporating more exercise into your daily routine.

4. Aerobics

Aerobics refers to an aerobic exercise routine that involves rhythmic movements performed with the use of our own body weight and muscle power in order to burn calories. The benefits of aerobics are improved posture, body tone, better cardiovascular health and increased flexibility and energy levels.

Dirty vs Clean Fast

To get the full benefit of the "clean" fast, eat whole foods and clear liquids with some basic supplements like vitamins. Outside of the fast, the dieter is allowed to eat food as long as it is "clean" and does not make them sick or cause any negative side effects. The dirty fasts, on the other hand, are a collection of pre-packaged foods that typically include meat, eggs, butter, and other unhealthy fats and sugars intended to put your body into a negative energy state.

For women over 50 who want to lose weight, keep a healthy weight, and improve their overall health, a week of clean and dirty fasts is perfect. The advantages of going the green route outweigh the drawbacks. If you're trying to lose weight or keep a healthy lifestyle, a week of dirty and clean fasting might be helpful.

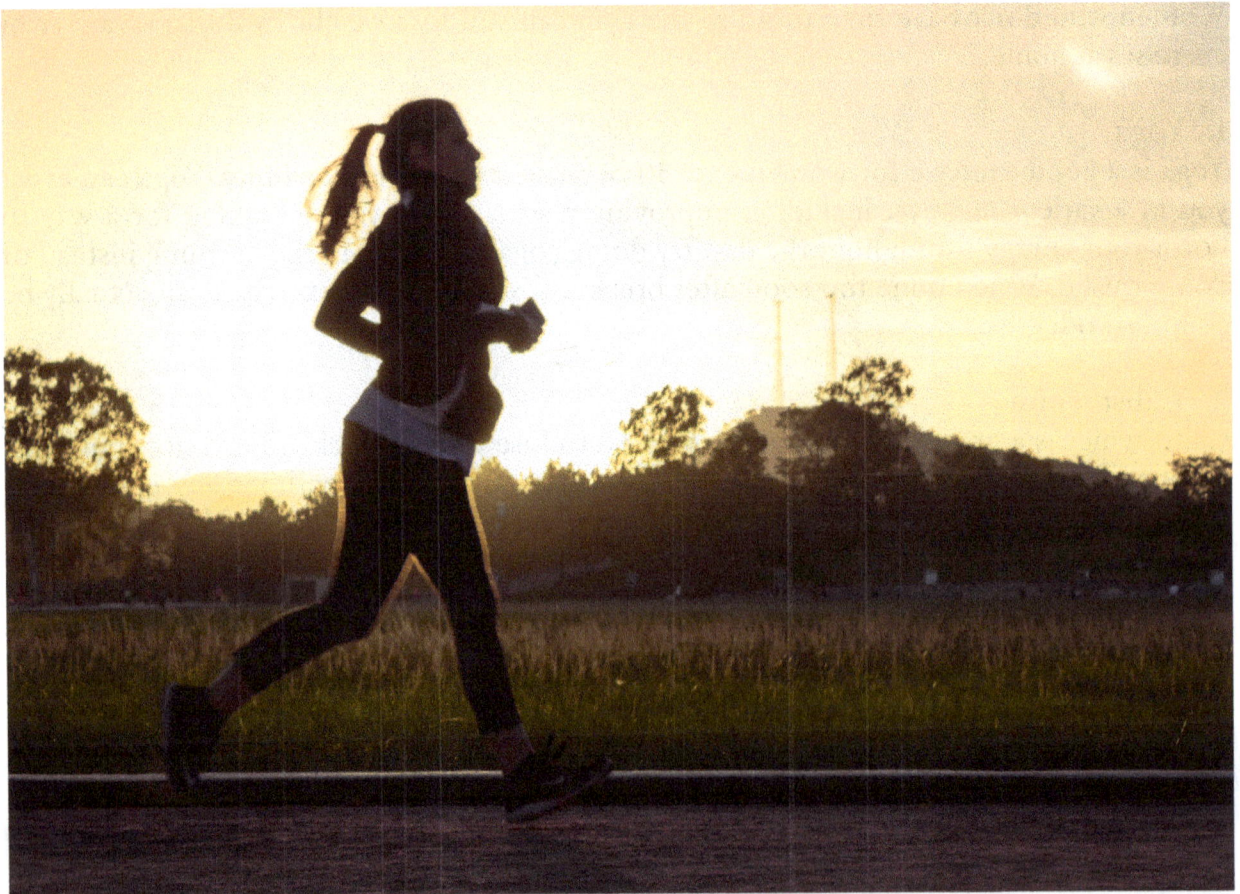

CHAPTER 4

A Successful Change
Starts In Your Mind

When it comes to one's ultimate health and desire to achieve the targets, controlling appetite, and keeping healthy food is important. Intermittent fasting will help you accomplish this, but although certain individuals can fast with very little problem for long stretches, some people can find it a bit more challenging, particularly when they first start.

There is a set of ideas to help you out that one can use to get the best results and make the ride a little smoother.

Start the Fast After Dinner
One of the best advice one can offer is when you do regular, or weekly fasting is to begin the fast after dinner. Using this ensures you're going to be sleeping for a good portion of the fasting time. Especially when using a daily fasting method like 16:8

Eat More Satisfying Meals
The type of food one consumes affects their willingness to both the urge to complete the fast and what you crave to eat after the fast. Too much salty and sugary foods with making you hungrier rather than consume meals that are homey satisfying and will help you lose weight

- Morning eggs or oats porridge
- A healthy lunch of chicken breast, baked sweet potato, and veggies.
- After the workout, drink a protein milkshake.
- Then you end the day in the evening with an equally impressive dinner.

Control Your Appetite
Without question, while fasting, hunger pangs can set in from start to end. The trick as this

occurs is to curb your appetite, and with Zero-calorie beverages that help provide satiety and hold hunger at bay before it's time to break the fast, the perfect way to do this is. Examples of food to consume are

- Sparkling water
- Water
- Black tea
- Black coffee
- Green tea
- Herbal teas and other zero-calorie unsweetened drinks

Stay Busy

Boredom is the main threat. It is the invisible assassin who, bit by bit, creeps in to ruin the progress, breaking you down steadily and dragging you downwards. For a second, think about it. How often boredom has caused you to consume more than you can, intend to, or even know that you are. Hence try to plan your day.

Stick to A Routine

Start and break your fast each day at regular times. Consuming a diet weekly where you finish similar items per day. Meal prepping in advance. Planning allows things easier to adhere to the IF schedule, so you eliminate the uncertainty and second-guess the process until you learn what works for you and commit to it every day. Follow-through is what one has to do.

Give Yourself Time to Adjust

When one first starts intermittent fasting, odds are you're going to mess up a couple of times; this is both OK and natural. It's just normal to have hunger pangs. This doesn't mean that you have to give up or that it's not going to be effective for you. Alternatively, it's a chance to learn, to ask whether or how you messed up, and take action to deter it from occurring again.

Enjoy Yourself

Let yourself enjoy the process. No one starts at the pro level, so you should go out with your friends and attend those birthday parties as well.

Chapter 5

What to Do and Don't Do while Fasting

How to Stay Healthy After 50

Lack of Sleep is Bad for Your Health
Sleeping is an essential part of human life and getting the amount of sleep a body needs to run well will help you in intermittent fasting, keeping you active.

Stay Hydrated
Drink 250ml of more water on an empty stomach. This will help you support your energy level and help you digest well for the day. Don't drink unhealthy juices on an empty stomach. It might give you terrible gas trouble and an enlarged tummy.

Keep a Food Diary
Keeping a food journal will help you with watching your calories. Furthermore, you will see any weight reduction all through your fast. This will help you with coordinating eating affinities and developing a step-by-step plan as demonstrated by the prerequisites and increase your benefits.

Cut Down on Sugar
Excessive intake of sugar will harm your body in all the ways possible and all your hard work will be in vain. You can eat sweet fruits and vegetables if you have a sweet tooth.

Eat Healthily
Abstain from eating foods bad for you after a fast. Healthy meals ought to be the center of consideration. They will assist you with getting the vital supplements, for example, nutrients, to give you more energy during the fasting time frame.

Avoid Stress

Whenever we begin something new, especially if it is related to our body, we need to consider the possible stress it may cause. Stressing out about it might make it worse. Keep calm, do your thing, and do not stress out. Remember that fasting implies not eating foods for some time. When fasting, be consistent with yourself and try not to eat before the named time. It will guarantee that you lose the greatest amount of weight and get the most benefits from intermittent fasting in solid terms.

COMMON INTERMITTENT FASTING MISTAKES TO AVOID

The results of intermittent fasting vary from one person to the other, but overall, every individual should be able to reap some benefits from the fasting. The key is doing it right and doing it consistently. Here are some common mistakes that could compromise your outcome:

Starting with an Extreme Plan

Now that you have found a fasting plan that sounds just perfect for your needs, don't you just want to jump in there with all your enthusiasm and, well, kick the hell out of it? You must be already imagining your new look after shedding those extra pounds. Can the fasting start already? Well, not so fast. Start with skipping single meals. Or avoiding snacks. Once your body gets used to short fasts, you can proceed to as far as your body can take, within reasonable limits. Go slow on exercising as well during the fasting phase, at least in the initial weeks, as it could cause adrenal fatigue.

Quitting too soon

Have you been fasting for a paltry one week and have already decided that it is too hard? Are you struggling with the hunger pangs, cravings, mood swings, low energy levels and so on? Well, such a reaction should be anticipated. The first couple of weeks can be harsh as the body adjusts to the reduced calorie intake. You will be hungry, irritable and exhausted. Still, you will be required to remain consistent. Even if you cannot feel it, the body is adapting to the changes. Hang in there; things will get better with time.

'Feasting' too much

Some quarters refer to intermittent fasting as alternating phases of fasting and feasting. This largely suggests that as soon as the clock hits the last minute of fast time, you dig right into a large savory meal, the kind that you end with a loud satisfied belch. Ideally, there should be nothing wrong with this approach, after all, you've successfully made it through your fasting window.

But remember your main goal here is to burn fat and lose weight. That only works if you have fewer calories going in compared to those going out. The larger your meal, the higher the number of calories that you're introducing into the body.

Insufficient Calories

While some will binge eat to make up for the 'lost time,' others will eat very little, fearing to turn back the gains already made. This results in inadequate calories, yet these calories are required to fuel the body to perform its functions optimally. With insufficient nutrients, you're likely to experience mood swings, irritability, fatigue, and low energy levels. Your day-to-day life will be compromised, and you'll be less productive. Intermittent fasting should make your life better, not worse. Eating enough will allow you to remain active and proceed efficiently with your fasting plan.

Wrong Food Choices

Go for healthy, wholesome foods that will nourish your body with all groups of nutrients. Let your meal contain adequate portions of vegetables, protein, good fats and complex carbs. You may have heard that intermittent fasting works well with a low-carb diet. That's right, but it's a low-carb, not a no-carb diet. Some people try to accelerate weight loss by eliminating all carbs. Remember carbs supply us with calories to fuel the body. Include a portion of healthy starch on your plate, going for brown unprocessed options where applicable.

Insufficient Fluids

Staying hydrated makes your fast more tolerable. It gives you a full feeling and keeps hunger pangs at bay. Fasting also breaks down the damaged components in the body, and the water helps flush them out as toxins.

You can also sip tea or coffee, with no milk or sugar added. Coffee has been known to contain compounds which further accelerate the burning of fat. Green tea also has similar properties. You can experiment with different flavors of tea or coffee to get a taste that appeals to you. As long as they don't contain any calories, they're good to go.

Over-concentrating on the Eating Window

If you can't take your eyes off the clock, you're not doing it right. You can't spend the fasting phase obsessing over food, thinking of what and how much you'll eat when it's finally time. In fact, the more you think about food, the hungrier you get. That hunger you feel every 5 hours or so is emotional hunger. It is clock hunger, which you'll feel around the normal mealtimes. Real hunger mostly checks in when you've been fasting for 16 hours onwards. Get your mind off food and concentrate on something else. If you're at home and keep circling the kitchen, leave and go somewhere else. Go to the library, for shopping (not for food of course), to the park or attend to your errands. Food is so much easier to keep away from when it's out of sight.

Wrong Plan

We have already been through the various fasting plans available, as well as the factors to consider when choosing a fasting plan. That should guide you to comfortable fasting. How do you know that the plan you are following is not the best one for you? To begin with, the entire process becomes a major strain. You struggle with hunger, fatigue, mood swings, and low energy levels. Your performance in your duties is affected, and you dread the next fast. And even after all the struggle, there's hardly any significant result to show for it. Go back and study the plans and choose one that better suits your lifestyle.

Stress

If you're under a great deal of stress, chances are you'll struggle through the fast. Stress causes hormone imbalances leaving you struggling with hunger pangs when you should have been fasting comfortably. Stress eating is common, characterized by cravings which drive you towards fatty and sugary foods. It also interferes with sleep, and fasting is even harder when you're not well rested. If you've already attempted the fast and have fallen into any of these mistakes, as many often do, you can correct yourself and proceed. If you're just starting out, you now know the pitfalls to avoid. The key is to keep learning and improving, and the results will be a testament to your effort.

MANAGING HUNGER

When it comes to dealing with starvation, the best thing to do is imagine it as a wave passing over you. The buildup to that wave can be excruciating at times, but it will finally crest and crash, passing entirely over and through you. Instead, keep yourself busy and take a few sips of a soda while you wait. These hunger pangs will become more bearable and not as overwhelming as they were at first. By the third day, you should have vastly improved your ability to deal with these hunger pangs.

DRINKING COFFEE

Coffee will be extremely beneficial to you during your fast. Coffee will help you get through the first few days of fasting, but it will eventually wear off. Remember, no sugar or milk with your coffee! That just adds more calories to your diet and aggravates your hunger.

CHEAT MEALS

Many people would overeat during the first few days of fasting. They may even believe they have broken the fast and begin thinking about food, so it is best to avoid these chronic overeaters from the start. The best way to deal with this is to indulge in a cheat meal on the first day of your fast. If you've never fasted before, this may appear to be a bad idea. It's important to remember that the hunger will pass, and you'll forget about the delicious meals that will give you energy for the next few days.

APPLE CIDER VINEGAR

When it comes to breaking your fast, apple cider vinegar can be a great ally. Drinking apple cider vinegar will not only make you physically feel better, but it will also improve your mental health. Mixing apple cider vinegar with the warm water is the best way to consume it. Remember to dilute it in equal parts if you continue to do this during your fasting time.

Consuming Snacks

It may have been tempting to overeat while fasting, so resist the temptation. If you eat when you shouldn't and restart your fast, it will be extremely difficult to break the fast without feeling extremely hungry and potentially suffering further harm. Take a short break after each meal, go out with friends, or spend time with family members to keep your mind and body busy.

Using Supplements with Intermittent Fasting

Fish Oil

Fasting requires the use of fish oil, which is an important supplement. Fish oil has been shown to be useful whether you are fasting or not, so it is best to take it on a daily basis. Taking fish oil will help keep your cholesterol from rising during this difficult time in your life. The fish oil in your body will assist you in dealing with the high levels of insulin and triglycerides associated with fasting.

Protein Powder

When you're trying to lose weight, you can also add protein powder to your diet. Many people will only eat proteins for the first few days of fasting, but you can also add protein powder to your diet when you want to break your fast. Protein powder is not something you can consume every day during the fasting period. Eating protein every day is highly recommended for those who are completely committed to fasting.

Calcium and Vitamin D

When fasting, calcium and vitamin D are also useful supplements to take. Calcium aids in the regulation of blood sugar, while vitamin D aids in the proper functioning of your entire body. Calcium may also help to prevent osteoporosis, a condition that causes bones to deteriorate. If your bones are weak or you are predisposed to osteoporosis, you can take this supplement on a daily basis.

B Vitamins

When it comes to vitamins, B vitamins should be taken as a combination rather than as individual supplements. B vitamins are responsible for the production of energy and fatty acids in your body. If this is the only supplement you take while fasting, you're missing out on one of the most important benefits of fasting. This combination will help you gain energy while also improving your hormonal balance.

Creatine

Creatine mimics and is made from the same substance found naturally in your body. Creatine is a substance that boosts energy and endurance, so consider including it in your supplement regimen. Creatine can help you feel great while fasting and also help you lose fat while building muscle mass.

Green Tea

Green tea is another effective supplement to take while fasting. Green tea will lift your spirits and make you feel wonderful. It will also assist you in losing a significant amount of weight while remaining healthy and feeling great. Green tea often includes antioxidants, which can aid in your body's recovery from fasting.

OMAD (ONE MEAL A DAY) AND INTERMITTENT FASTING

OMAD is nothing more than a fasting technique. Instead of eating once every three days, you will fast every other day. This can be accomplished by combining eating and not eating, or by skipping meals entirely. The amount of body fat lost on any diet is determined by how much you eat and how many calories you burn each day through exercise. Intermittent fasting keeps daily calorie intake to 600-800 while still allowing for some exercise.

KETO DIET AND INTERMITTENT FASTING

A perfect diet can be created by combining fasting and the ketogenic diet. Fasting reduces insulin production, which means you won't experience catabolism or muscle tissue breakdown while on a ketogenic diet. The ketogenic diet reduces blood glucose levels, but if you eat too much protein, your blood sugar will spike due to a lack of insulin to regulate it.

One of the reasons people make this diet mistake is that they use too much protein to replace carbs. When following this diet, it is critical that you do not exceed 1 gram of protein per pound of body weight. Some people can eat more than this, but you should not exceed 1 gram per pound because it can interrupt ketone production, which is required for fat burning. To keep this diet working, you'll need to keep track of your ketone levels as well as your blood glucose levels.

You must eat at least 100 grams of fat per day if you are fasting on this diet. While the OMAD diet does include fat, the two diets can be combined for a successful weight loss plan. It is also critical that your daily protein intake is less than 30 grams and your daily carbohydrate intake is less than 30 grams.

AUTOPHAGY

What is Autophagy?
Autophagy refers to the process by which your cells eat themselves. Cells are actively removing obsolete components. When you eat a meal, the leftovers are broken down into smaller molecules and transported to different cellular compartments known as autophagosomes. When food is not present in the cell, the contents of these autophagosomes are free to be used for energy by other cellular components or even discarded entirely. Consider this to be a recycling process that happens in all of your body's cells.

What are the benefits of Autophagy and Intermittent Fasting?
Autophagy aids in the protection against oxidative stress and the reduction of inflammation. Harmful compounds and bacteria can be removed from your body during this process. It aids in the development of muscle tissue, which is another way to burn calories during the day. The ketogenic diet has many advantages, but because of its high fat content, it can cause oxidative stress. Autophagy is a process by which your cells defend themselves from free radical damage inside the body.

HOW DOES THE OMAD DIET AND AUTOPHAGY WORK?
When you eat a meal, your body is continuously attempting to break it down. Even when you are sleeping, your cells are breaking down the calories from the preceding meal. The OMAD diet will provide your body with plenty of fat and protein to work on while you sleep. This helps to reduce some of the oxidative stress caused by eating a lot of fat while fasting.

INTERMITTENT FASTING FOR VEGANS
Vegans often have questions about how they can maintain an intermittent fasting plan while not eating any animal products. The good news is that there are vegan meat substitutes such as seitan, tofu, and jackfruit.

If you dislike eating animal products, you can still follow the OMAD diet. Simply make sure your meals contain at least 15 grams of fat and 20 grams of protein. Other vegan diets may include meals containing as little as 10 grams of fat and 20 grams of protein. Because protein is essential, plant-based foods can provide a good balance of fat and protein. When following an intermittent fasting schedule, vegetable oils such as canola, peanut, olive, and flaxseed oil are excellent sources of fat. Consume plenty of healthy fats to aid in weight loss. Other foods that can help you lose weight on a vegan diet include eggplant, aubergine (eggplant), pumpkin, onions, kale, spinach, broccoli, and salad greens.

SWITCH FROM CLEAN TO DIRTY FASTING
The clean eating diet, like any other diet or nutrition plan, must be cycled. You should reintroduce the dirty fast into your diet after 5-10 days or so. Remember that the best

thing about intermittent fasting is that it eliminates the need for calorie counting. With intermittent fasting, you can eat whatever you want and still lose weight. The only thing to be concerned about after a fast is what to eat.

The best foods are those that are high in protein and fiber. Low sugar fruits, greens, vegetables, legumes, grains, and, of course, healthy fats like avocados, olive oil, and coconut oil are all options. However, don't start eating sugar or animal products because they will not benefit your body in any way.

When is it appropriate to switch from clean to dirty fasting? When following a diet or nutrition plan, it's easy to lose track of time, but if you don't keep track of your fasting cycles, you'll soon find yourself cheating on the clean eating diet. Fast for 5-10 days, followed by a few days of eating only whole foods. When that time is up, you can resume the clean fasting diet by eating only fruits and vegetables for the next few days.

NUTRIENT-DENSE DIET WHEN FASTING
When following the OMAD diet, make sure your meals are nutrient-dense. Fruits and vegetables can be a good source of vitamins, minerals, and antioxidants. When following the OMAD diet, fiber-rich foods should be prioritized. This will assist you in incorporating more foods into your meals in order to make them more attractive. It is critical to be aware of your daily macronutrient intake. It is best to eat 1 gram of protein per pound of body weight per day to maintain good health.

YOU DO NOT NEED TO COUNT CALORIES
One of the most common issues with many people is that they become disheartened simply because they have to cut calories. The best thing about intermittent fasting is that you don't have to reduce your calorie intake at all. You don't even need to count calories to see if you're eating more or less. You must consume the amount of food that will satisfy you. Excess calories don't matter much in intermittent fasting as long as you eat healthy foods.

It is critical that your meals contain all of the macro-ingredients in the proper proportions. This means that if you're trying to lose weight. Then your carbs should be high-fat, low-carb, and medium-protein. You don't need to be alarmed about the fact that eating fat is recommended for weight loss because we'll explain why.

Fat, protein, and carbs all play important roles in your well-being. You will still feel drained of energy if you do not eat them in proper proportion. As a result, it is important for your meals to contain a good balance of the three.

BREAKING OUT OF AN INTERMITTENT FASTING PLATEAU

You will begin to feel better than you have ever felt before if you stick to your intermittent fasting schedule. You will not experience overeating or other unfavorable food-related problems. The only remaining problem is the desire to lose weight.

It is vital that you make some dietary changes if you want to continue seeing results. As far as possible, avoid sugary and processed foods. Fast food contains unnecessary fats and sugars that can sabotage your weight loss efforts.

Make your meals more interesting by including a variety of fruits and vegetables.

Fiber should be a part of every meal. Avoid using supplements to lose weight because they may jeopardize your efforts and make you feel worse rather than better. Eat as many healthy fats as you can because they will keep you whole. Keep in mind that you are fasting when you sleep, so make sure your meals are high in healthy fat.

When you wake up in the morning, your body is most likely depleted of energy. If you consume sugar or fiber, both of which are fast-digesting carbs, your energy levels will spike and then crash. This will make it difficult to concentrate and may even leave you feeling drained of energy.

What you should do is as follows:

It's true! Drink coffee! A single cup of coffee will assist you in getting out of bed in the morning. This is due to the fact that it will stimulate your nervous system. People who are tired often crave sugar or carbohydrates, so coffee will help you overcome these cravings without jeopardizing your diet.

Drink water: If your meals are high in fat, you won't need any extra water in your system to keep you satiated. Having said that, you should still drink at least 8 glasses of water per day because it has other advantages. Among the advantages are improved digestion and the prevention of headaches and constipation.

Consume more protein: Aim for 1 gram of protein per pound of body weight. This is a simple way to increase your levels of essential amino acids and aid in weight loss without feeling hungry or tired.

Consume plenty of veggies: Fruits and vegetables help to build muscle mass. Having said that, you should eat a large part of these meals every day because they are high in vitamins, minerals, antioxidants, and fiber.

BURN YOUR FAT NOT YOUR MUSCLES!

When you fast, your body uses its own fat stores for energy, which causes you to lose weight. If you want to gain muscle, you must stop eating protein and start eating carbs.

Keep in mind that autophagy happens in your body when you sleep. This is why, when fasting, nutrient-dense meals are important because they aid in the process.

To ensure that your body burns fat, you must balance a fair number of calories from fat, carbs, and protein while fasting. Simply eating enough protein will help you achieve this.

Eating perfectly balanced, nutrient-dense meals will help you feel full and not hungry throughout the day. This will allow you to lose weight without feeling hungry. It is also critical to consume plenty of healthy fats because they are an excellent source of energy.

The most effective way to gain muscle mass is to combine strength training with proper nutrition. The best diet for muscle mass includes eating adequate protein and carbohydrates while reducing your fat intake. Your body will burn more fat when building and repairing muscle tissue if you do this.

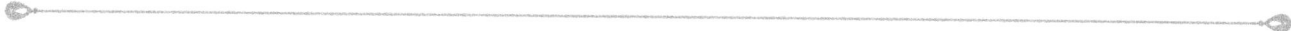

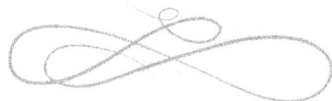

CHAPTER 6

Lunch Recipes

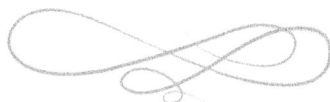

I. Sesame-Seared Salmon

Ingredients:
- 4 wild salmon fillets (about 1lb.)
- 1½ tbsps. Sesame seeds
- 2 tbsps. Toasted sesame oil
- 1½ tbsps. Avocado oil
- 1 tsp. sea salt

Preparation time: 5 min.
Cooking time: 10 min.
Servings: 4

Calories: 198
Protein: 12g
Fat: 5g

Directions:
1. Using a paper towel or a clean kitchen towel, pat the fillets to dry. Brush each with a tablespoon of sesame oil and season with a half teaspoon of salt.
2. Place a large skillet over medium-high heat and drizzle with avocado oil. Once the oil is hot, add the salmon fillets with the flesh side down. Cook for about 3 minutes and flip. Cook the skin side for an additional 3-4 minutes, without overcooking it.
3. Remove the pan from the heat and brush with the remaining sesame oil. Season with the remaining salt and sprinkle with sesame seeds. Best served with green salad.

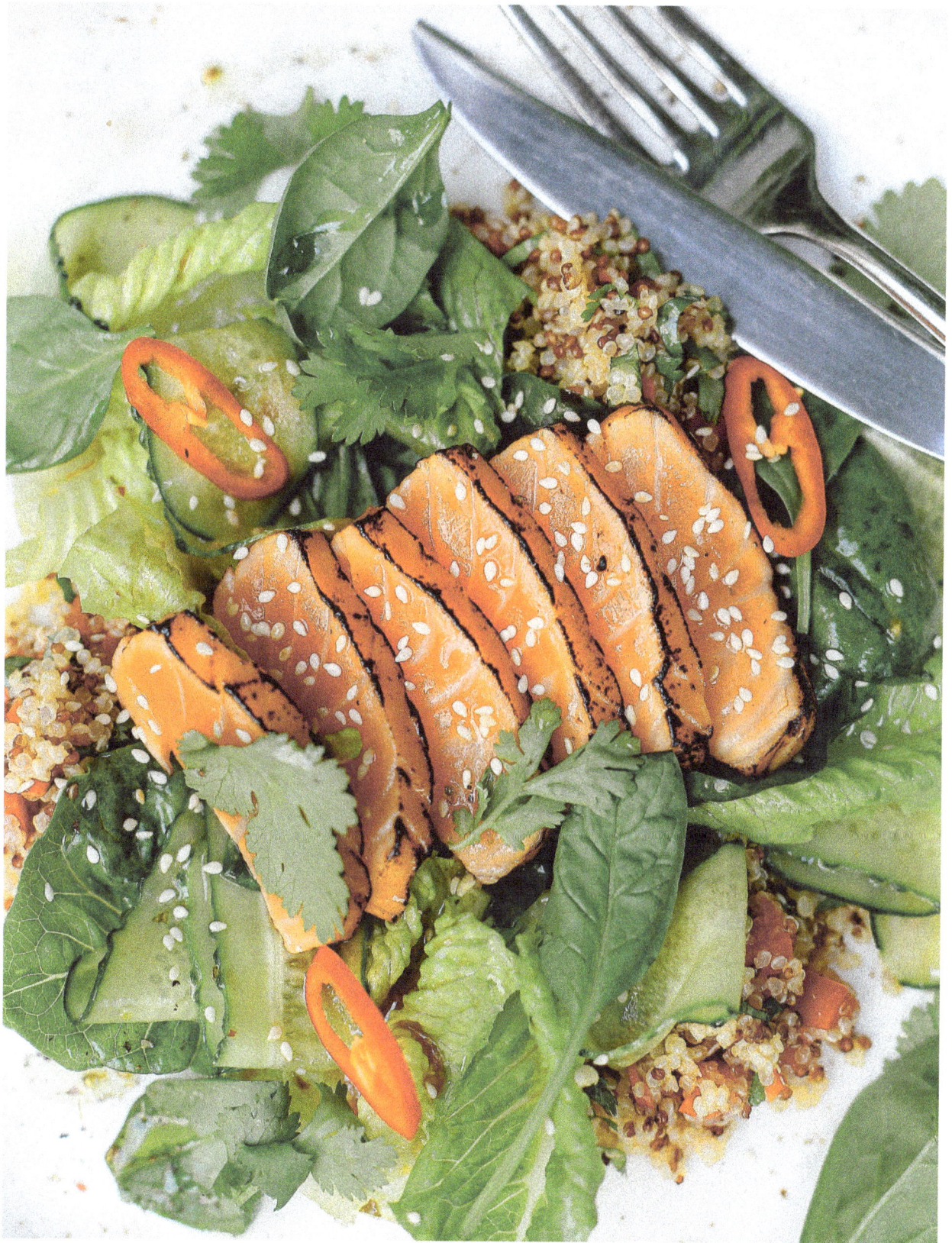

2. TURKEY WALNUT SALAD

INGREDIENTS:

- 0.25 cup Chopped walnuts
- 1 Chopped celery
- 0.5 pc. Chopped yellow onion
- 8 oz. Minced turkey
- Pepper
- Salt
- 2 tsp. Parsley
- 1 tsp. Lemon juice
- 1 tbsp. Dijon mustard
- 2 tbsps. Greek yogurt
- 2 tbsps. Mayo
- 3 tbsps. Dried cranberries

Preparation time: 10 min.
Cooking time: 20 min.

Calories: 390
Protein: 4g
Fat: 56g

DIRECTIONS:

1. Take out a bowl and combine the cranberries, walnuts, celery, onion, and turkey.
2. In another bowl, combine the pepper, salt, parsley, lemon juice, mustard, Greek yogurt, and mayo.
3. Combine both bowls together and toss well to mix evenly before serving.

---

3. SPINACH SAMOSA

INGREDIENTS:

- 1 ½ cups of almond flour
- ½ teaspoon baking soda
- 1 teaspoon garam masala
- 1 teaspoon coriander, chopped
- ¼ cup green peas
- ½ teaspoon sesame seeds
- ¼ cup potatoes, boiled, small chunks
- 2 tablespoons olive oil
- ¾ cup boiled and blended spinach puree
- Salt and chili powder to taste

AIR FRYER REQUIRED

Preparation time: 15 min.
Cooking time: 15 min.
Servings: 2

Calories: 254
Protein: 12.2g
Fat: 10.2g

DIRECTIONS:

1. In a bowl, mix baking soda, salt, and flour to make the dough. Add 1 tablespoon of oil. Add the spinach puree and mix until the dough is smooth.
2. Place in the fridge for 20 minutes.
3. In the pan add one tablespoon of oil, then add potatoes, peas and cook for 5 minutes. Add the sesame seeds, garam masala, coriander, and stir.
4. Knead the dough and make the small ball using a rolling pin. Form balls, make into cone shapes, which are then filled with stuffing that is not yet fully cooked. Make sure flour sheets are well sealed.
5. Preheat the air fryer to 390° F. Place samosa in the air fryer basket and cook for 10 minutes.

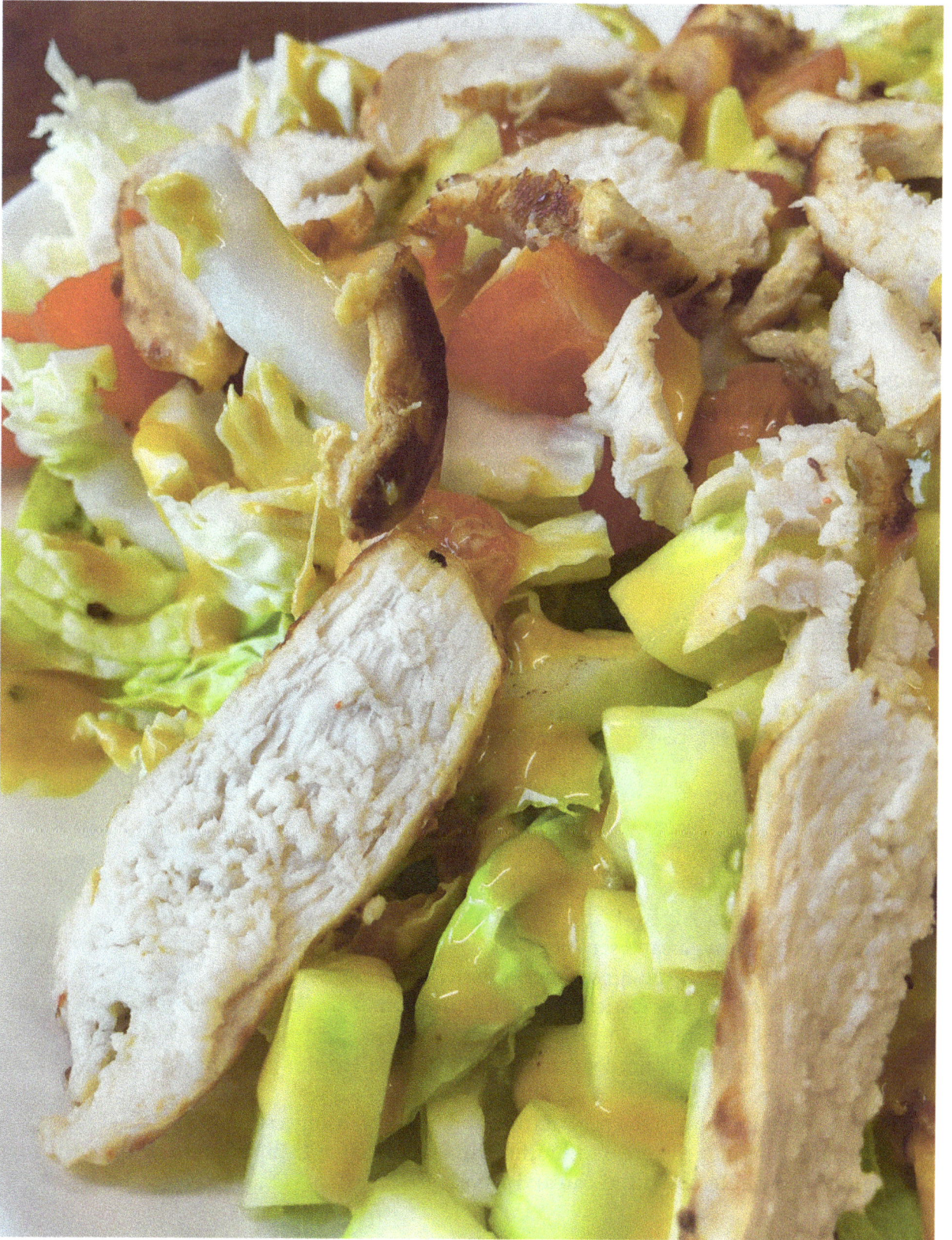

4. MINI THAI LAMB SALAD BITES

INGREDIENTS:

- 1 large cucumber, cut into 0.39-inch-thick diagonal rounds
- 0.55 lb. (250g) Lamb Blackstrap
- 3/4 cup Cherry Tomatoes, quartered
- 1/3 cup fresh mint, loosely packed
- 1/3 cup fresh coriander, loosely packed
- 1/4 small red onion, finely diced
- 1 tsp. fish sauce
- Juice of 1 lime
- Coconut oil

Preparation time: 10 min.
Cooking time: 8 min.
Servings: 15

Calories: 58
Protein: 2g
Fat: 5g

DIRECTIONS:

1. Place pan over medium heat and heat oil. Cook the lamb for 4 minutes on each side. Remove from heat and let it rest.
2. In a mixing bowl, toss the onions, tomatoes, mint, coriander, fish sauce, and lime juice.
3. Cut the lamb into thin strips and add to the salad bowl. Toss to combine.
4. Spoon ample amount of mixture on each cucumber cut. Chill and serve.

5. BACON EGG & SAUSAGE CUPS

INGREDIENTS:

- 3 oz. breakfast sausages
- 2 slices bacon, chopped
- 4 large eggs
- 2 large green onions, chopped
- 1 oz. cheddar cheese, shredded
- 1 tbsp. coconut oil

Preparation time: 10 min.
Cooking time: 20 min.
Servings: 8

Calories: 100
Protein: 8g
Fat: 5g

DIRECTIONS:

1. Preheat the oven to 350°F.
2. Grease your muffin pan and set aside.
3. In a mixing bowl, beat the eggs together with the cheese. Set aside.
4. Brown the bacon in a non-stick skillet over medium heat. Add the crumbled sausage and cook until no longer pink.
5. Add the onion and cook until wilted. Remove the skillet from the heat and let it cool for a minute or two.
6. Add the meat mixture to the egg mixture and beat well using a spoon.
7. Scoop mixture into the greased muffin pan and bake for 15-20 minutes or until the tops begin to brown. Remove from pan and serve.

6. Easy Italian Zucchini Fritters

Ingredients:

- 4 cloves minced garlic
- 1 teaspoon sea salt
- 2 large eggs
- 2 teaspoons Italian seasoning
- 8 cups grated zucchini
- 1 cup parmesan cheese, grated
- Olive oil to fry with

Preparation time: 15 min.
Cooking time: 20 min.
Servings: 6

Calories: 127
Protein: 6g
Fat: 10g

Directions:

1. Place the zucchini and salt into a large colander and mix together. Drain over the sink for 10 minutes.
2. Wrap the zucchini in a kitchen towel. Squeeze and twist over the sink to drain as much water as possible.
3. Place the zucchini into a large bowl. Add remaining ingredients and stir them together.
4. Heat a generous amount of olive oil in a large skillet over medium-high heat for about 2 minutes. Spoon rounded tablespoonfuls (28 grams) of the batter onto the skillet and flatten to about 1/4 to 1/3 inch thick. Fry for about 2 minutes on each side until golden brown.
5. Serve with sour cream and parsley.

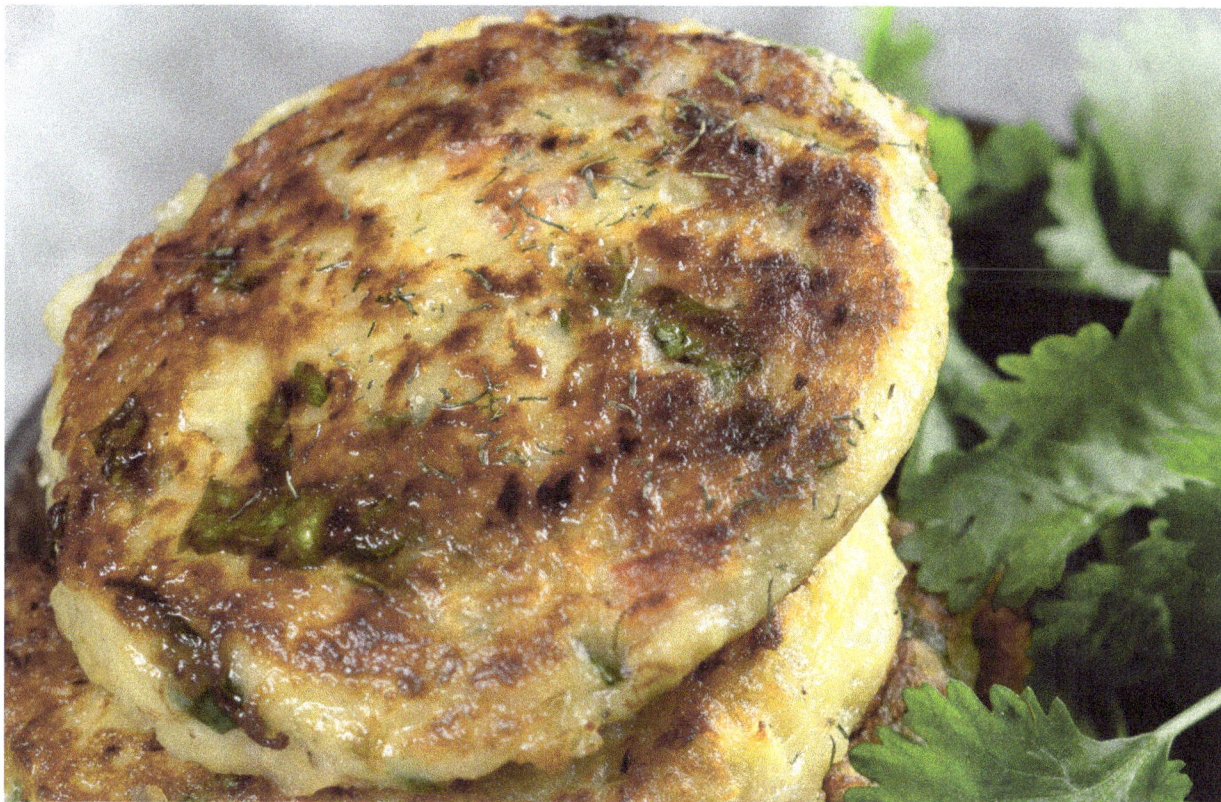

7. Smoked Salmon & Avocado Stacks

INGREDIENTS:

- ½ lb. smoked salmon, finely diced
- 1 ripe avocado, seed removed and diced
- 1 tbsp. chives, chopped
- Fresh or dried dill leaves
- 3 tsps. fresh lemon juice
- Black pepper, cracked

Preparation time: 15 min.
Cooking time: 0 min.
Servings: 6

Calories: 106
Protein: 12g
Fat: 5g

DIRECTIONS:

1. Combine salmon, chives, and a teaspoon of lemon juice in a small mixing bowl.
2. In another mixing bowl, toss the avocado, remaining lemon juice, and pepper.
3. Using a presentation ring, arrange the stacks on the serving plates. Arrange the avocado at the bottom and top it with the salmon mixture and gently press. Remove the mold and garnish the stack with dill leaves. Serve chilled.

8. Pasta Bolognese Soup

INGREDIENTS:

- 2 tsp olive oil
- 3 onions, chopped finely
- 2 carrots, peeled and chopped finely
- 2 celery stick, chopped finely
- 3 cloves of garlic, chopped finely
- 250g of lean steak/beef mince
- 500g pasta
- 1 tbsp vegetable stock
- 1 tsp paprika, smoked works well
- 4 pieces of thyme, fresh
- 100mg penne, whole meal
- 45g parmesan cheese, grated finely

Preparation time: 10 min.
Cooking time: 35 min.
Servings: 5

Calories: 182
Protein: 4g
Fat: 3g

DIRECTIONS:

1. Take a large pan and add the oil, heat over a medium heat
2. Add the onions and cook until translucent
3. Add the carrots, garlic, and the celery, cooking for 5 minutes
4. Add the mince to the pan and break it up well
5. Once the mince has browned, add the stock and the passata, adding 1 liter of hot water
6. Stir well and then add the thyme and paprika, combining once more
7. Add the lid to the pan and allow to simmer for 15 minutes
8. Add the penne and stir through, cooking for another 165 minutes
9. Add the cheese and stir
10. Serve in bowls whilst still warm

9. QUICK RATATOUILLE

INGREDIENTS:

- 2 onions, sliced
- 4 cloves of garlic, chopped very finely
- 0.5 cup olive oil
- 1 green pepper, cut into small pieces
- 1 red pepper, cut into small pieces
- 1 aubergine (eggplant), cut into cubes
- 4 zucchinis, cubed
- 8 tomatoes, seeded and chopped
- 1 tbsp basil, shredded. Fresh is best but if you have to go with dried, just use 1 tsp)
- 1.5 tsp salt
- A little black pepper

Preparation time: 10 min.
Cooking time: 12 min.
Servings: 4

Calories: 270
Protein: 8g
Fat: 6g

DIRECTIONS:

1. You will need a large and deep-frying pan or saucepan,
2. Add the oil and allow to reach a medium to high heat
3. Add the onions and the garlic and cook for a few minutes, until the onions are clear
4. Add the peppers, zucchini, and the aborigine (eggplant) and combine
5. Turn the heat down and play an over the pan, allowing it to simmer for around 10 minutes
6. Add the salt and pepper, as well as the tomatoes and stir well, covering the pan once more and allowing it to continue cooking for another 10 minutes
7. Take the lid off the pan and stir the mixture, allowing it to reduce
8. Add a little salt and pepper and serve whilst still warm. The mixture is done when it is blended well, but isn't particularly 'wet'

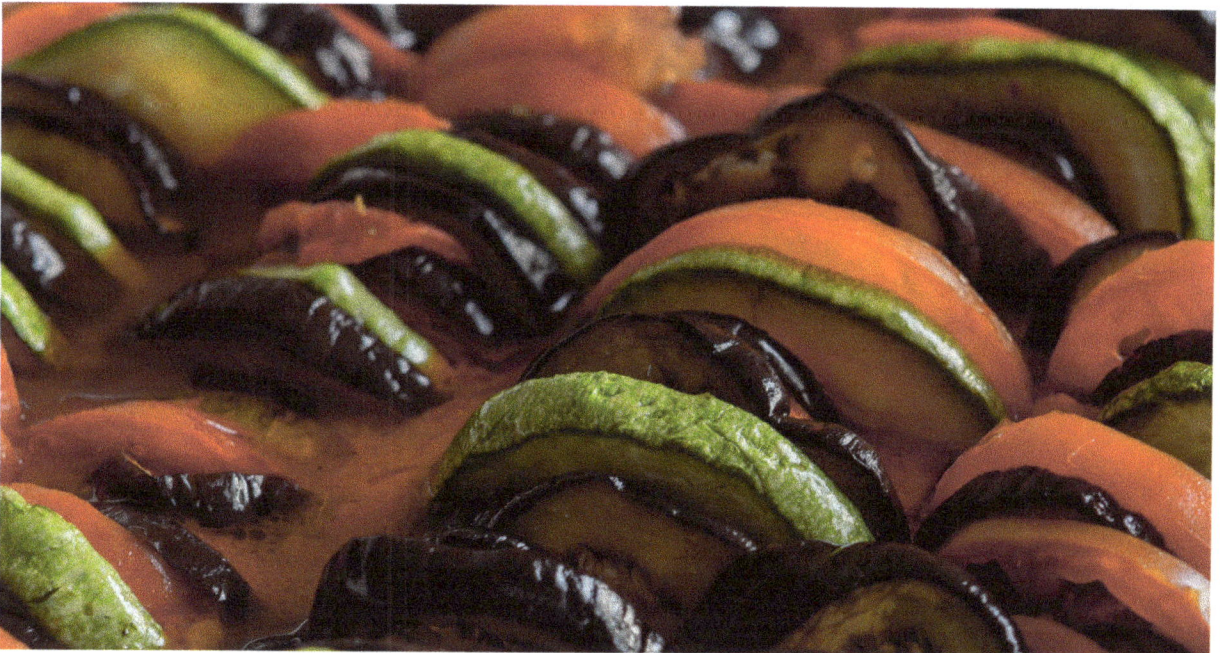

10. CRISPY HERB CAULIFLOWER FLORETS

INGREDIENTS:

- 1 egg, beaten
- 2 tablespoons parmesan cheese, grated
- 2 cups cauliflower florets, boiled
- ¼ cup almond flour
- 1 tablespoon olive oil
- Salt to taste
- ½ tablespoon mixed herbs
- ½ teaspoon chili powder
- ½ teaspoon garlic powder

AIR FRYER REQUIRED

Preparation time: 20 min.
Cooking time: 15 min.
Servings: 2

Calories: 253
Protein: 11.3g
Fat: 8.5g

DIRECTIONS:

1. In a bowl, combine garlic powder, breadcrumbs, chili powder, mixed herbs, salt, and cheese. Add olive oil to the breadcrumb mixture and mix well.
2. Place flour in a bowl and place the egg in another bowl. Dip the cauliflower florets into the beaten egg, then in flour, and coat with breadcrumbs.
3. Preheat your air fryer to 350° F. Place the coated cauliflower florets inside an air fryer basket and cook for 20 minutes.

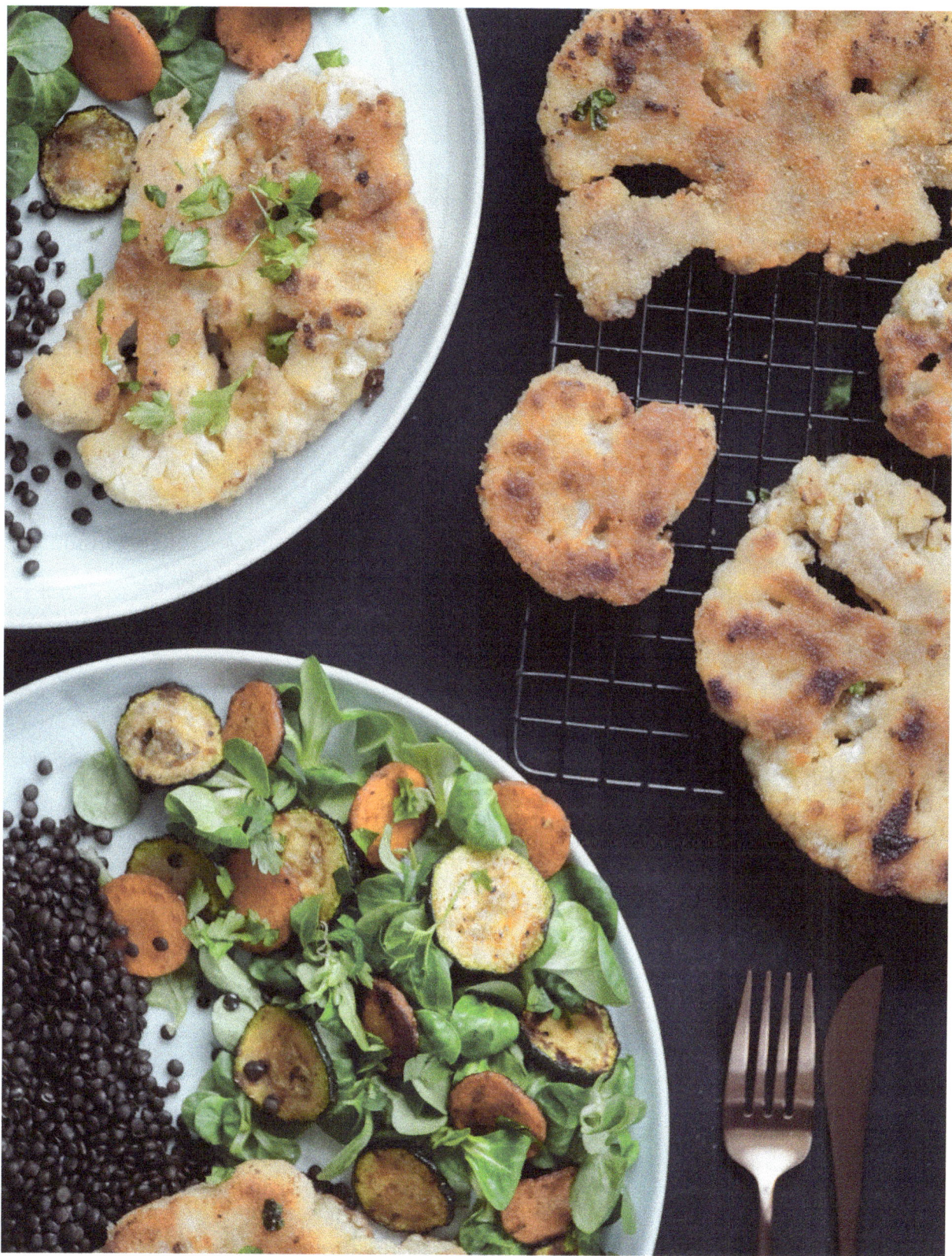

11. Honey Roasted Carrots

INGREDIENTS:

- 1 tablespoon honey
- Salt and pepper to taste
- 3 cups of baby carrots
- 1 tablespoon olive oil

AIR FRYER REQUIRED

Preparation time: 12 min.
Cooking time: 15 min.
Servings: 2

Calories: 257
Protein: 11.6g
Fat: 7.3g

DIRECTIONS:

1. In a mixing bowl, combine carrots, honey, and olive oil.
2. Season with salt and pepper.
3. Cook in an air fryer at 390° F for 12 minutes.

12. Low Carb Cabbage Bowl

INGREDIENTS:

- 2 tablespoons of olive oil
- ½ cup of chopped carrots
- ¼ cup of diced onions
- ½ tsp of salt
- ½ tsp of pepper
- 1 tsp of cumin
- ½ tsp of turmeric
- 1 cup of shredded cabbage
- 1 cup of chopped potatoes

Preparation time: 3 min.
Cooking time: 14 min.
Servings: 4

Calories: 327
Protein: 7g
Fat: 18g

DIRECTIONS:

1. Place a medium sized saucepan onto a burner set for high heat and add your 2 tablespoons of olive oil to the pan.
2. Next, add your ½ cup of chopped carrots, your ¼ cup of diced onions, your ½ tsp of salt, and your ½ tsp of pepper.
3. Stir and cook these ingredients for about 4 minutes before adding your cup of shredded cabbage, and your cup of chopped potatoes, followed by your tsp of cumin and your ½ tsp of turmeric.
4. Continue to stir and cook your ingredients for about 10 more minutes.
5. Turn the burner off, allow food to cool for a moment and serve.

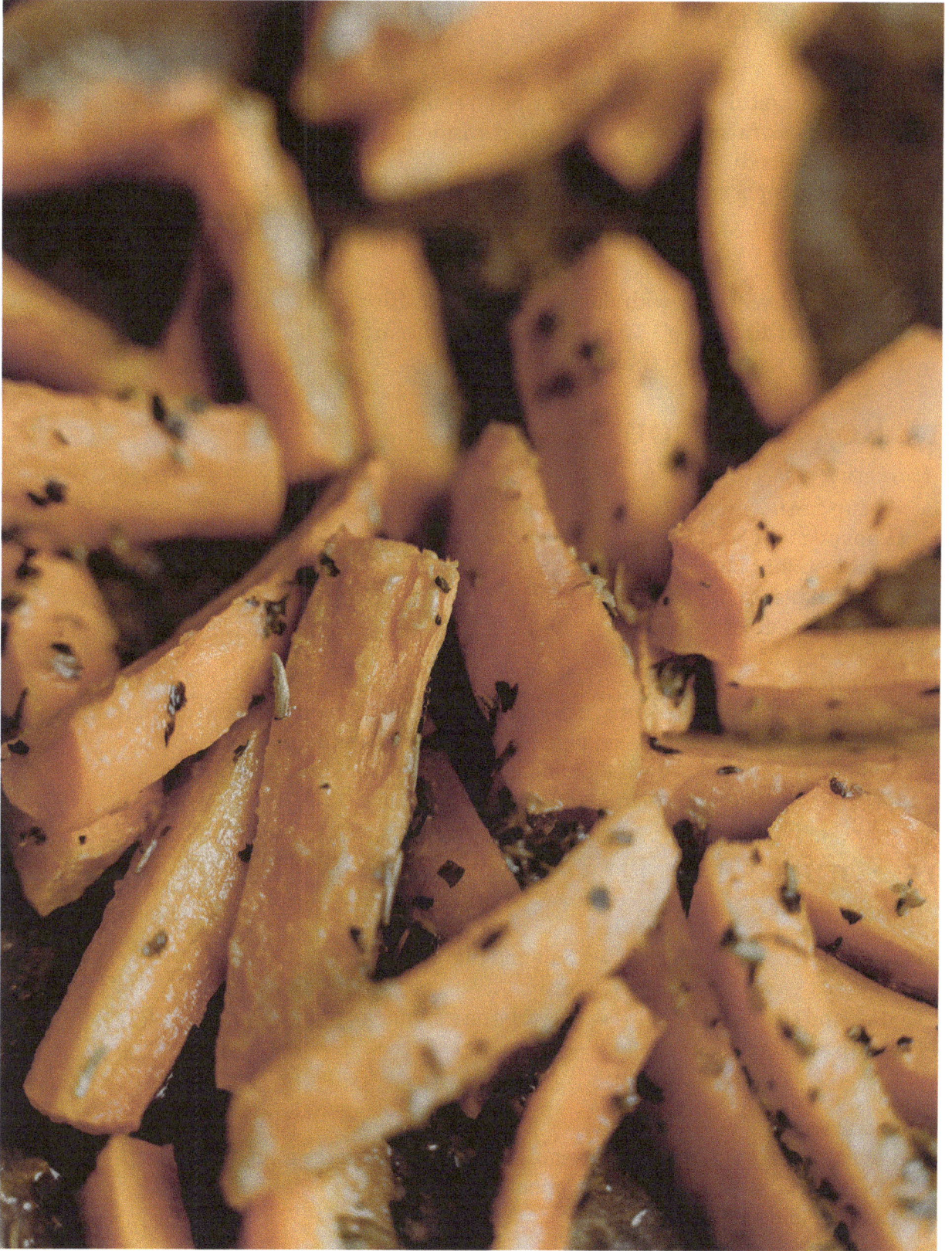

14. Tasty Tofu

INGREDIENTS:

- ¼ cup cornmeal
- 15 ounces extra firm tofu, drained, cubed
- Salt and pepper to taste
- 1 teaspoon chili flakes
- ¾ cup cornstarch

AIR FRYER REQUIRED

Preparation time: 12 min.
Cooking time: 15 min.
Servings: 4

Calories: 246
Protein: 11.2g
Fat: 7.6g

DIRECTIONS:

1. Line the air fryer basket with aluminum foil and brush with oil.
2. Preheat your air fryer to 370° F. Mix all ingredients in a bowl.
3. Place in the air fryer and cook for 12 minutes.

13. Roasted Trout

INGREDIENTS:

- ½ cup fresh lemon juice
- 1 pound trout fish fillets
- 4 tablespoons butter
- Salt and black pepper, to taste
- 1 teaspoon dried rosemary, crushed

Preparation time: 10 min.
Cooking time: 35 min.
Servings: 4

Calories: 349
Protein: 28.2g
Fat: 23.3g

DIRECTIONS:

1. Put ½ pound trout fillets in a dish and sprinkle with lemon juice and dried rosemary.
2. Season with salt and black pepper and transfer into a skillet.
3. Add butter and cook, covered on medium low heat for about 35 minutes.
4. Dish out the fillets in a platter and serve with a sauce.

15. Sour Cream Tilapia

INGREDIENTS:

- ¾ cup homemade chicken broth
- 1 pound tilapia fillets
- 1 cup sour cream
- Salt and black pepper, to taste
- 1 teaspoon cayenne pepper

Preparation time: 10 min.
Cooking time: 3 hours
Servings: 3

Calories: 300
Protein: 17.9g
Fat: 31.8g

DIRECTIONS:

1. Put tilapia fillets in the slow cooker along with the rest of the ingredients.
2. Cover the lid and cook on low for about 3 hours.
3. Dish out and serve hot.

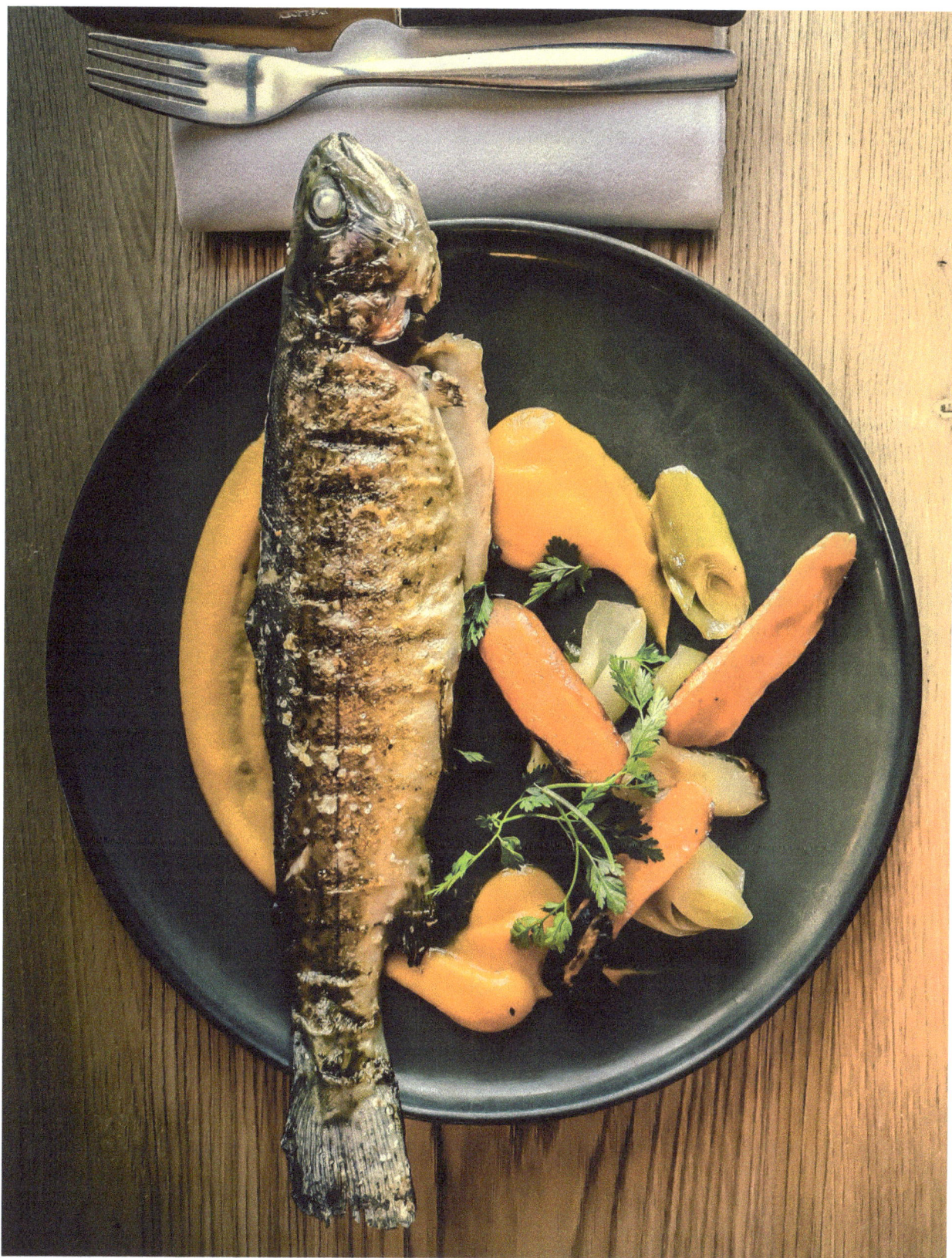

16. Instant Pot Teriyaki Chicken

INGREDIENTS:

- 1/2 cup soy sauce
- 1/2 cup water
- 1/2 cup brown sugar
- 2 tbsps. rice wine vinegar
- 1 tbsp. mirin (Japanese sweet wine)
- 1 tbsp. sake
- 1 tbsp. minced garlic
- 1 dash freshly cracked black pepper
- 1 lb. skinless, boneless chicken

PRESSURE COOKER REQUIRED

Preparation time: 5 min.
Cooking time: 35 min.
Servings: 4

Calories: 259
Protein: 24.3g
Fat: 2.3g

DIRECTIONS:

1. Combine soy sauce, brown sugar, water, rice wine vinegar, sake, mirin, pepper, and garlic in a bowl to prepare the sauce.
2. Put chicken in an electric pressure cooker (such as Instant Pot(R)). Pour the sauce over.
3. Close lid and lock. Set to Meat function, with the timer on to 12 minutes. Give 10-15 minutes for pressure to build.
4. Gently release pressure with the quick-release method according to manufacturer's Directions, for 5 minutes. Remove the lid. Insert the instant-read thermometer into the middle of the chicken and make sure to reach at least 165°F (74°C). If not hot enough, cook for 2-4 more minutes.
5. Take chicken out from the cooker. Shred or cut up. Mix with sauce from the pot.

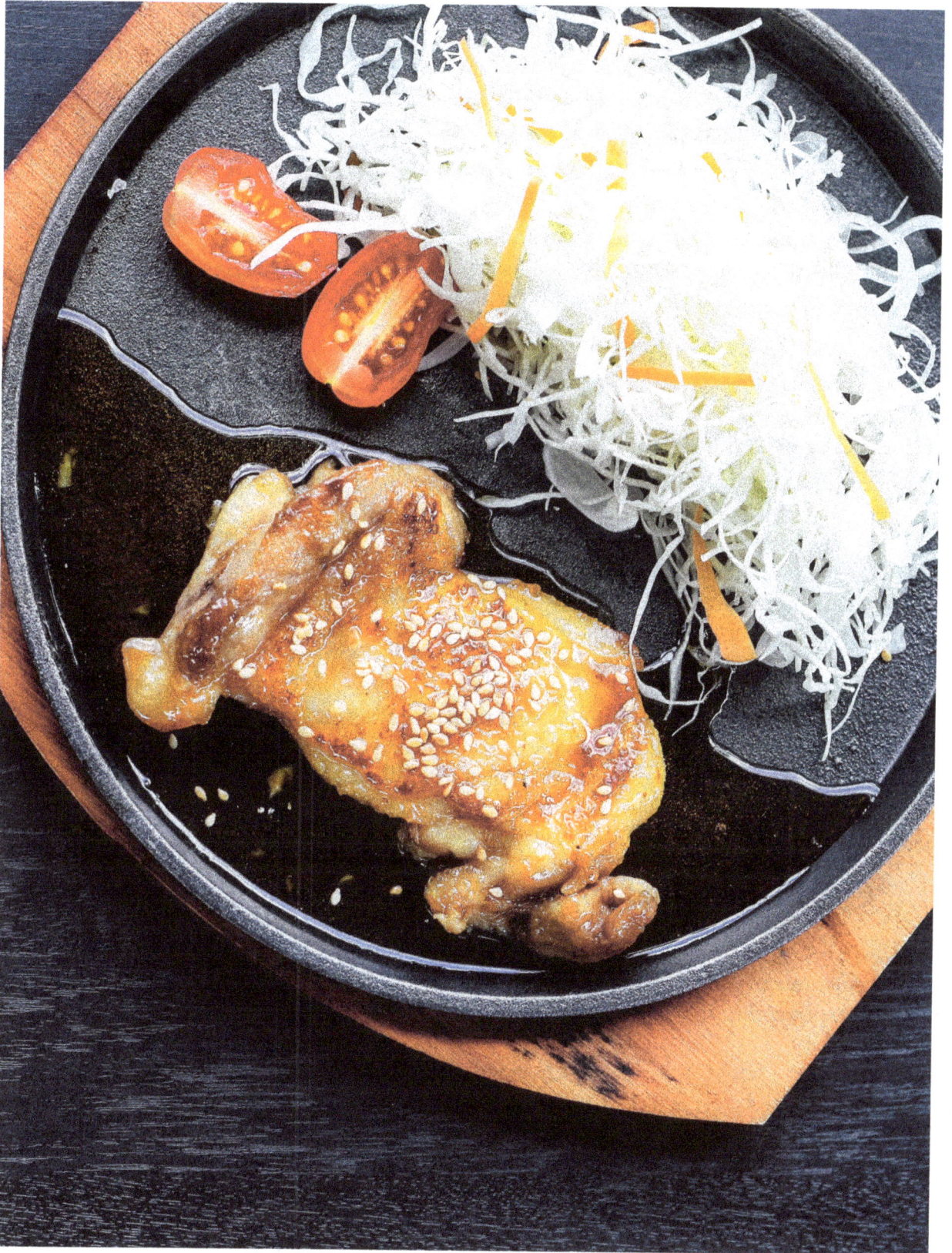

17. ROASTED CORN

INGREDIENTS:

- 4 ears of corn
- Salt and pepper to taste
- 3 teaspoons vegetable oil

DIRECTIONS:

1. Remove the husks from corn, wash and pat them dry.
2. Cut if needed to fit into an air fryer basket.
3. Drizzle with vegetable oil and season with salt and pepper.
4. Cook at 400 F for 10 minutes.

AIR FRYER REQUIRED

Preparation time: 10 min.
Cooking time: 15 min.
Servings: 8

Calories: 256
Protein: 9.4g
Fat: 9.2g

---

18. EGG & SAUSAGE CUPS

INGREDIENTS:

- 15 ounces black-eyed peas
- 1/8 teaspoon chipotle chili powder
- ¼ teaspoon salt
- ½ teaspoon chili powder
- 1/8 teaspoon black pepper

Preparation time: 10 min.
Cooking time: 15 min.
Servings: 6

Calories: 262
Protein: 9.4g
Fat: 9.2g

DIRECTIONS:

1. Rinse the beans well with running water then set aside.
2. In a large bowl, mix the spices until well combined. Add the peas to spices and mix.
3. Place the peas in the wire basket and cook for 10 minutes at 360° F.
4. Serve and enjoy!

---

19. SPICY NUTS BACON

INGREDIENTS:

- 2 cups mixed nuts
- 1 teaspoon chipotle chili powder
- 1 teaspoon salt
- 1 teaspoon pepper
- 1 tablespoon butter, melted
- 1 teaspoon ground cumin

AIR FRYER REQUIRED

Preparation time: 4 min.
Cooking time: 15 min.
Servings: 8

Calories: 252
Protein: 8.6g
Fat: 8.4g

DIRECTIONS:

1. In a bowl, add all ingredients and toss to coat.
2. Preheat your air fryer to 350° F for 5 minutes.
3. Add mixed nuts into the air fryer basket and roast for 4 minutes.

20. Garlic Butter Beef Steak

INGREDIENTS:

- 1 lb. beef sirloin steaks
- ½ cup red wine
- 4 tbsps. unsalted butter
- 2 tbsps. fresh parsley, finely chopped
- 4 medium garlic cloves, peeled and minced
- Fine sea salt and freshly cracked black pepper

PRESSURE COOKER REQUIRED

Preparation time: 5 min.
Cooking time: 15 min.
Servings: 2

Calories: 337
Protein: 34.5g
Fat: 18.7g

DIRECTIONS:

1. Season the beef steaks with sea salt and freshly cracked black pepper.
2. On the Instant Pot, press "Sauté" and add the butter. Once melted, add the beef steaks and sear for 2 minutes per side or until brown.
3. Pour in the red wine and fresh parsley. Cover and cook for 12 minutes on high pressure. When done, release the pressure naturally and carefully remove the lid.
4. Top the steak with the butter sauce. Serve and enjoy!

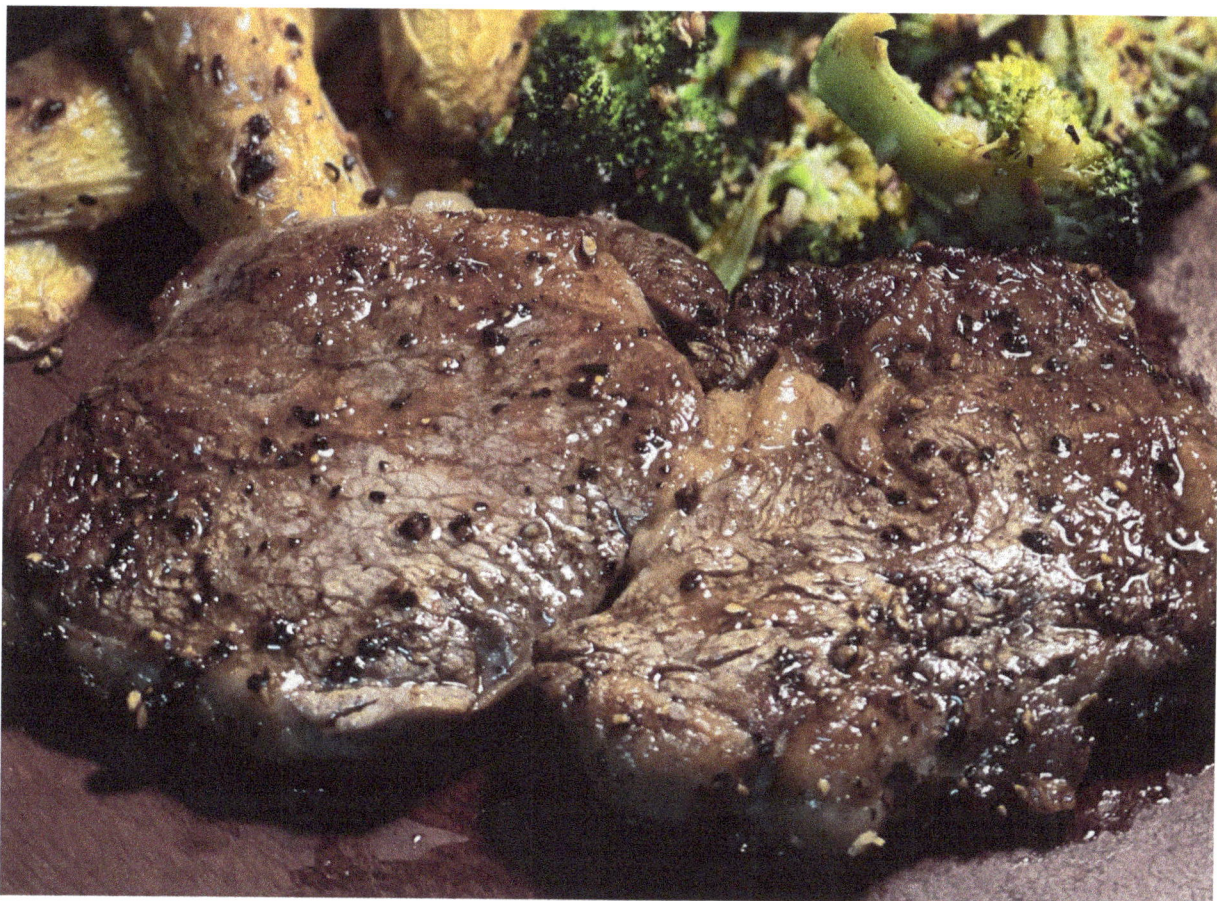

21. LEAN GREEN SOUP

INGREDIENTS:

- 500 ml vegetable stock
- 1 tablespoon of coconut oil
- 1 tablespoon of minced garlic
- 2 tablespoons of water
- 1 tsp of coriander
- 1 tsp of turmeric
- ½ cup of chopped broccoli
- ½ cup of chopped kale
- ½ cup of chopped parsley

Preparation time: 3 min.
Cooking time: 9 min.
Servings: 4

Calories: 182
Protein: 10g
Fat: 8g

DIRECTIONS:

1. Add your tablespoon of coconut oil to a saucepan followed by your tablespoon of minced garlic, your tsp of coriander, and your tsp of turmeric.
2. Set the burner on high and add 2 tablespoons of water to the mix.
3. Stir ingredients together as they cook over the next 2 minutes.
4. Now add your 500 ml vegetable stock followed by your ½ cup of chopped broccoli, your ½ cup of chopped kale, and your ½ cup of chopped parsley.
5. Stir everything together well and allow to cook for another 7 minutes.
6. Allow to cool slightly, and serve when ready

22. PORTOBELLO MUSHROOM FAJITA WRAPS

INGREDIENTS:

- 3 corn tortillas
- 1 tablespoon of chopped jalapenos
- 2 tablespoons of olive oil
- 1 cup of chopped portobello mushrooms
- ¼ cup of chopped onions
- ¼ cup of chopped bell peppers
- 1 tablespoon of chopped garlic
- 1 tsp of cumin
- 1 tsp of smoked paprika
- ¼ tsp of salt

PRESSURE COOKER REQUIRED

Preparation time: 10 min.
Cooking time: 15 min.
Servings: 3

Calories: 207
Protein: 7g
Fat: 2g

DIRECTIONS:

1. Get out a large pan and place it onto a burner set for high heat before adding your tablespoon of chopped jalapenos, your ¼ cup of chopped onions, your ¼ cup of chopped bell peppers, your tsp of cumin, your tsp of smoked paprika, and your tablespoon of chopped garlic.
2. Stir and cook all of your ingredients together for about 2 minutes.
3. After this, add your cup of chopped mushrooms.
4. Continue to stir and cook your ingredients over the next 10 minutes.
5. Evenly distribute your cooked ingredients into your tortillas and wrap them up.
6. This dish is ready to eat!

23. Teriyaki Salmon

Ingredients:

- 3 tbsps. lime juice
- 2 tbsps. olive oil
- 2 tbsps. reduced-sodium teriyaki sauce
- 1 tbsp. balsamic vinegar
- 1 tbsp. Dijon mustard
- 1 tsp. garlic powder
- 6 drops hot pepper sauce
- 6 uncooked jumbo salmon

Preparation time: 15 min.
Cooking time: 5 min.
Servings: 2

Calories: 93
Protein: 13g
Fat: 4g

Directions:

1. Mix together all ingredients except the salmon in a big zip-lock plastic bag, then put in the shrimp. Seal the zip lock bag and turn to coat the salmon. Keep in the fridge for an hour and occasionally turn.
2. Drain the marinated salmon and discard marinade. Broil the salmon 4 inches from heat for 3 to 4 minutes per side or until the salmon turn pink in color.

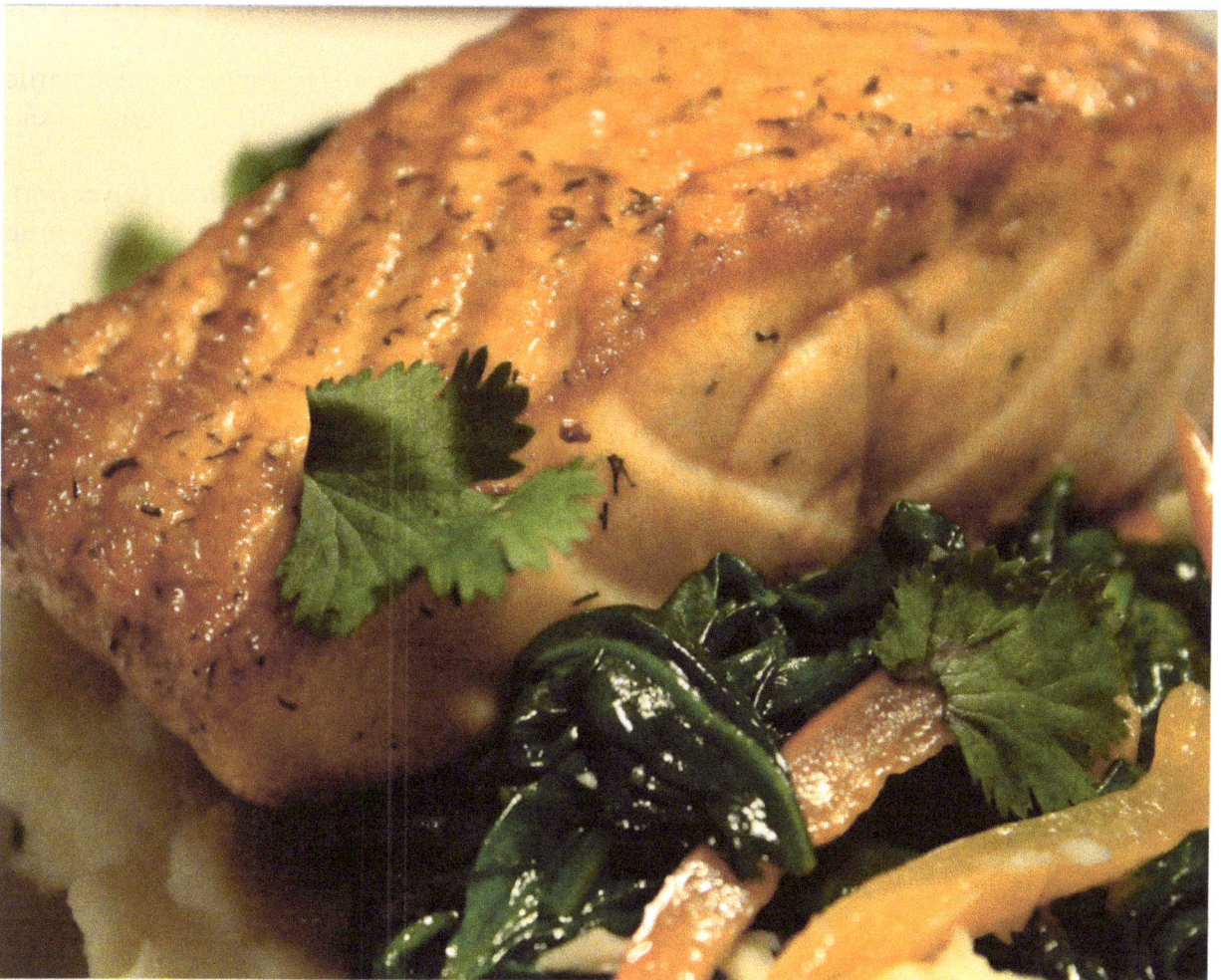

24. EGGPLANT PARMESAN PANINI

INGREDIENTS:

- 1 medium eggplant, cut into ½ inch slices
- ½ cup mayonnaise
- 2 tablespoons milk
- Black pepper to taste
- ½ teaspoon garlic powder
- ½ teaspoon onion powder
- 1 tablespoon dried parsley
- ½ teaspoon Italian seasoning
- ½ cup breadcrumbs
- Sea salt to taste
- Fresh basil, chopped for garnishing
- ¾ cup tomato sauce
- 2 tablespoons parmesan, grated cheese
- 2 cups grated mozzarella cheese
- 2 tablespoons olive oil
- 4 slices artisan Italian bread
- Cooking spray

AIR FRYER REQUIRED

Preparation time: 25 min.
Cooking time: 15 min.
Servings: 2

Calories: 267
Protein: 11.3g
Fat: 8.5g

DIRECTIONS:

1. Cover both sides of eggplant with salt. Place them between sheets of paper towels. Set aside for 30 minutes to get rid of excess moisture.
2. In a mixing bowl, combine Italian seasoning, breadcrumbs, parsley, onion powder, garlic powder and season with salt and pepper. In another small bowl, whisk mayonnaise and milk until smooth.
3. Preheat your air fryer to 400° F. Remove the excess salt from eggplant slices. Cover both sides of eggplant with mayonnaise mixture. Press the eggplant slices into the breadcrumb mixture. Use cooking spray on both sides of eggplant slices.
4. Air fry slices in batches for 15 minutes, turning over when halfway done. Each bread slice must be greased with olive oil.
5. On a cutting board, place two slices of bread with oiled sides down. Layer mozzarella cheese and grated parmesan cheese. Place eggplant on cheese. Cover with tomato sauce and add remaining mozzarella and parmesan cheeses.
6. Garnish with chopped fresh basil. Put the second slice of bread oiled side up on top. Take preheated Panini press and place sandwiches on it. Close the lid and cook for 10 minutes.
7. Slice panini into halves and serve.

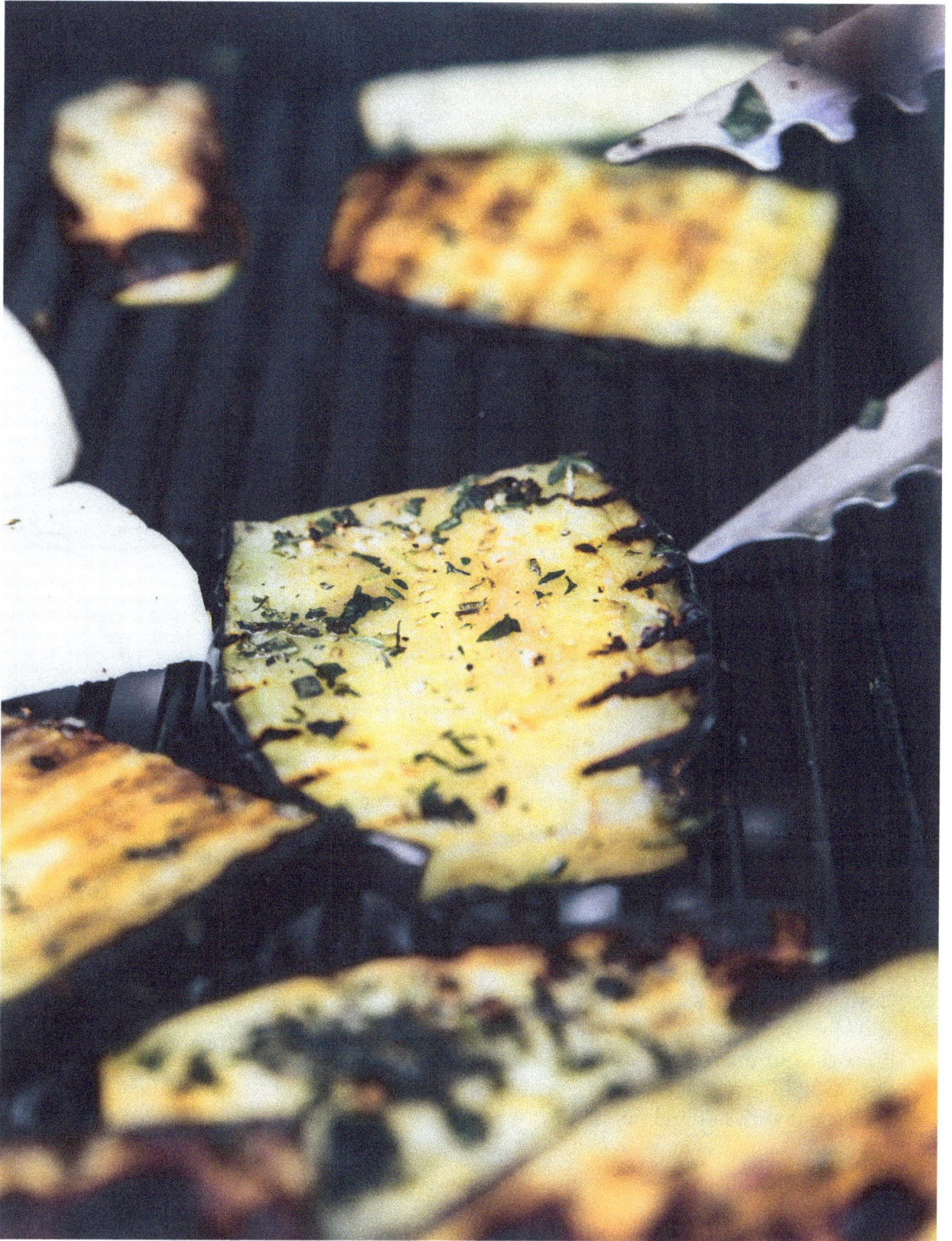

25. GARLIC BUTTER SALMON

INGREDIENTS:

- Kosher salt and black pepper, to taste
- 1 pound (3 pounds) salmon fillet, skin removed
- 4 tablespoons butter, melted
- 2 garlic cloves, minced
- ¼ cup parmesan cheese, freshly grated

Preparation time: 10 min.
Cooking time: 30 min.
Servings: 8

Calories: 172
Protein: 12.3g
Fat: 15.6g

DIRECTIONS:
1. Preheat the oven to 3500F and lightly grease a large baking sheet.
2. Season the salmon with salt and black pepper and transfer to the baking sheet.
3. Mix together butter, garlic and parmesan cheese in a small bowl.
4. Marinate salmon in this mixture for about 1 hour.
5. Transfer to the oven and bake for about 25 minutes.
6. Additionally, broil for about 2 minutes until the top becomes lightly golden.
7. Dish out onto a platter and serve hot.

26. GROUND BEEF AND CAULIFLOWER HASH

INGREDIENTS:

- 1 large zucchini, sliced
- 1 green pepper, sliced
- 1 large parsnip, peeled and cubed
- Salt and black pepper to taste
- 2 tablespoons honey
- 2 cloves garlic, crushed
- 1 teaspoon mixed herbs
- 1 teaspoon mustard
- 6 tablespoons olive oil, divided
- 4 cherry tomatoes
- 1 medium carrot, peeled and cubed

AIR FRYER REQUIRED

Preparation time: 20 min.
Cooking time: 15 min.
Servings: 4

Calories: 262
Protein: 11.3g
Fat: 7.4g

DIRECTIONS:
1. Add the zucchini, green pepper, parsnip, cherry tomatoes, carrot to the bottom of the air fryer.
2. Cover ingredients with 3 tablespoons of oil and adjust the time to 15 minutes. Cook at 360° F.
3. Prepare your marinade by combining remaining ingredients in an air fryer safe baking dish. Combine marinade and vegetables in a baking dish and stir well.
4. Sprinkle it with salt and pepper. Cook it at 390° F for 5 minutes.

27. Garlic Shrimp with Goat Cheese

Ingredients:

- 4 tablespoons herbed butter
- Salt and black pepper, to taste
- 1 pound large raw shrimp
- 4 ounces goat cheese
- 4 garlic cloves, chopped

Preparation time: 30 min.
Cooking time: 20 min.
Servings: 4

Calories: 294
Protein: 15g
Fat: 35.8g

Directions:

1. Preheat the oven to 3750F and grease a baking dish.
2. Mix together herbed butter, garlic, raw shrimp, salt and black pepper in a bowl.
3. Put the marinated shrimp on the baking dish and top with the shredded cheese.
4. Place in the oven and bake for about 25 minutes.
5. Take the shrimp out and serve hot.

28. Tilapia with Herbed Butter

Ingredients:

- 2 pounds tilapia fillets
- 12 garlic cloves, chopped finely
- 6 green broccoli, chopped
- 2 cups herbed butter
- Salt and black pepper, to taste

Pressure Cooker Required

Preparation time: 35 min.
Cooking time: 25 min.
Servings: 6

Calories: 281
Protein: 10.4g
Fat: 38.7g

Directions:

1. Season the tilapia fillets with salt and black pepper.
2. Put the seasoned tilapia along with all other ingredients in an Instant Pot and mix well.
3. Cover the lid and cook on High Pressure for about 25 minutes.
4. Dish out on a platter and serve hot.

30. Low Carb Cabbage Bowl

INGREDIENTS:

- 2 tablespoons of olive oil
- ½ cup of chopped carrots
- ¼ cup of diced onions
- ½ tsp of salt
- ½ tsp of pepper
- 1 tsp of cumin
- ½ tsp of turmeric
- 1 cup of shredded cabbage
- 1 cup of chopped potatoes

Preparation time: 3 min.
Cooking time: 14 min.
Servings: 4

Calories: 327
Protein: 7g
Fat: 18g

DIRECTIONS:

1. Place a medium sized saucepan onto a burner set for high heat and add your 2 tablespoons of olive oil to the pan.
2. Next, add your ½ cup of chopped carrots, your ¼ cup of diced onions, your ½ tsp of salt, and your ½ tsp of pepper.
3. Stir and cook these ingredients for about 4 minutes before adding your cup of shredded cabbage, and your cup of chopped potatoes, followed by your tsp of cumin and your ½ tsp of turmeric.
4. Continue to stir and cook your ingredients for about 10 more minutes.
5. Turn the burner off, allow food to cool for a moment and serve.

29. Mahi Stew

INGREDIENTS:

- 2 tablespoons butter
- 2 pounds Mahi fillets, cubed
- 1 onion, chopped
- Salt and black pepper, to taste
- 2 cups homemade fish broth

PRESSURE COOKER REQUIRED

Preparation time: 15 min.
Cooking time: 30 min.
Servings: 3

Calories: 398
Protein: 12.5g
Fat: 62.3g

DIRECTIONS:

1. Season the Mahi fillets with salt and black pepper.
2. Heat butter in a pressure cooker and add onion.
3. Sauté for about 3 minutes and stir in the seasoned Mahi fillets and fish broth.
4. Lock the lid and cook on High Pressure for about 30 minutes.
5. Naturally release the pressure and dish out to serve hot.

31. PORK CARNITAS

INGREDIENTS:

- Pepper
- 0.25 tsp. Salt
- 0.5 tbsp. Dark molasses
- 0.5 tbsp. Orange juice
- 1 tbsp. Brown sugar
- 1 Minced garlic clove
- 0.5 lb. Pork tenderloin

Preparation time: 10 min.
Cooking time: 50 min.

Calories: 294
Protein: 12g
Fat: 45g

DIRECTIONS:

1. Rinse off the pork tenderloin and blot it down with some paper towels. Slice thinly and then set it aside.
2. Place a skillet on a flame or burner set to high, and then heat it up for about a minute. Once the skillet is hot, add the pork tenderloin. Cook these for about 4 minutes until the pork is tender and cooked throughout.
3. Drain out the oil before stirring in the pepper, salt, molasses, orange juice, and brown sugar.
4. Stir this around and simmer until your sauce is thick. Turn off the heat and let it stand for a few minutes to thicken before serving.

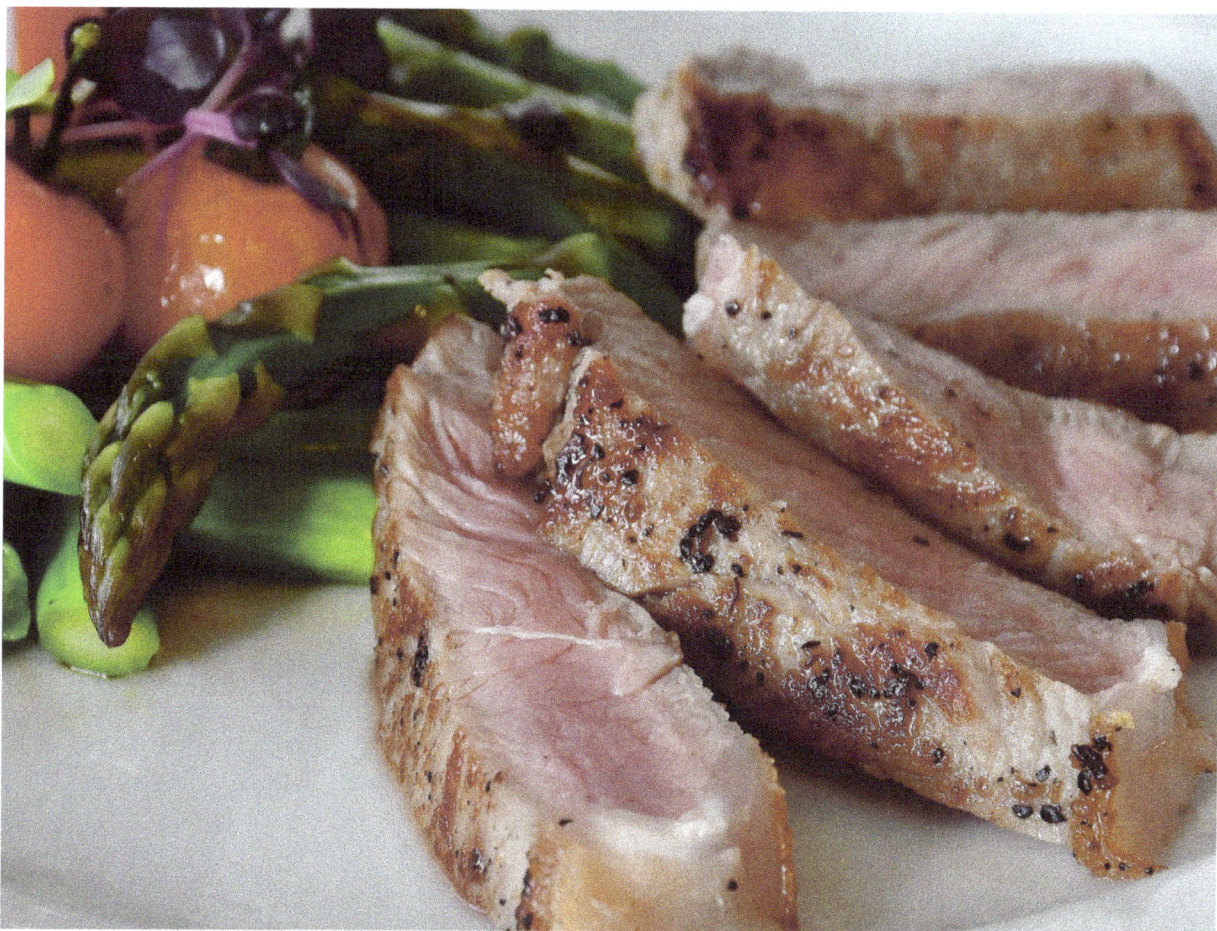

32. GRILLED PROSCIUTTO WRAPPED ASPARAGUS

INGREDIENTS:

- 16 asparagus spears, rimmed at the ends
- 4 slices Prosciutto
- Olive oil for greasing
- Kosher salt for tasting
- Black pepper for tasting

Preparation time: 5 min.
Cooking time: 10 min.
Servings: 4

Calories: 50
Protein: 4g
Fat: 2.5g

DIRECTIONS:

1. Cut each piece of prosciutto into 4 pieces and wrap each piece around the center of each spear.
2. Spritz with olive oil, season the asparagus tips with a pinch of salt and season the rest with black pepper.
3. Light the grill over light heat, when hot clean and oil the grates.
4. Grill the asparagus 5 to 6 minutes, covered on low turning every few minutes

33. SOUR FISH WITH HERBED BUTTER

INGREDIENTS:

- 2 tablespoons herbed butter
- 3 cod fillets
- 1 tablespoon vinegar
- Salt and black pepper, to taste
- ½ tablespoon lemon pepper seasoning

Preparation time: 45 min.
Cooking time: 30 min.
Servings: 3

Calories: 234
Protein: 11.8g
Fat: 31.5g

DIRECTIONS:

1. Preheat the oven to 3750F and grease a baking tray.
2. Mix together cod fillets, vinegar, lemon pepper seasoning, salt and black pepper in a bowl.
3. Marinate for about 3 hours and then arrange on the baking tray.
4. Transfer into the oven and bake for about 30 minutes.
5. Remove from the oven and serve with herbed butter.

34. SPICY OVEN BAKED CHICKEN

INGREDIENTS:

- 4 tablespoons of fat-free buttermilk
- 2 tablespoons of spicy brown mustard
- 2 lean chicken breasts
- ¼ cup of whole wheat breadcrumbs
- ¼ cup chopped walnuts
- 1 tablespoon of chopped rosemary
- ¼ tsp of salt
- ½ tsp of pepper
- ½ tsp of cayenne pepper
- 2 tablespoons of honey

Preparation time: 10 min.
Cooking time: 23 min.
Servings: 4

Calories: 248
Protein: 27g
Fat: 2g

DIRECTIONS:

1. Set your oven for 425 degrees.
2. While your oven warms up, get out a medium sized mixing bowl and add your 4 tablespoons of fat-free buttermilk and your 2 tablespoons of spicy brown mustard.
3. Now place each chicken breast into the bowl, and turn them over in the mixture, until they are thoroughly coated.
4. Next, place a frying pan onto a burner set for high heat and add your ¼ cup of wheat breadcrumbs to the pan, followed by your ¼ cup of chopped walnuts, your 1 tablespoon of chopped rosemary, your ¼ tsp of salt, your ½ tsp of pepper, and your ½ tsp of cayenne pepper and stir everything together well as they cook over the next 2 to 3 minutes before turning the burner off.
5. Now place your buttermilk coated chicken into the pan and flip it around in the cooked breadcrumb ingredients until they are thoroughly coated with it as well.
6. Place your breadcrumb coated chicken breasts in an oven safe dish and cook for about 20 minutes.
7. Serve when ready.

35. Cod Coconut Curry

Ingredients:

- 1 onion, chopped
- 2 pounds cod
- 1 cup dry coconut, chopped
- Salt and black pepper, to taste
- 1 cup fresh lemon juice

Directions:

1. Put the cod along with all other ingredients in a pressure cooker.
2. Add 2 cups of water and cover the lid.
3. Cook on High Pressure for about 25 minutes and naturally release the pressure.
4. Open the lid and dish out the curry to serve hot.

Pressure Cooker required

Preparation time: 35 min.
Cooking time: 25 min.
Servings: 6

Calories: 223
Protein: 35.5g
Fat: 6.1g

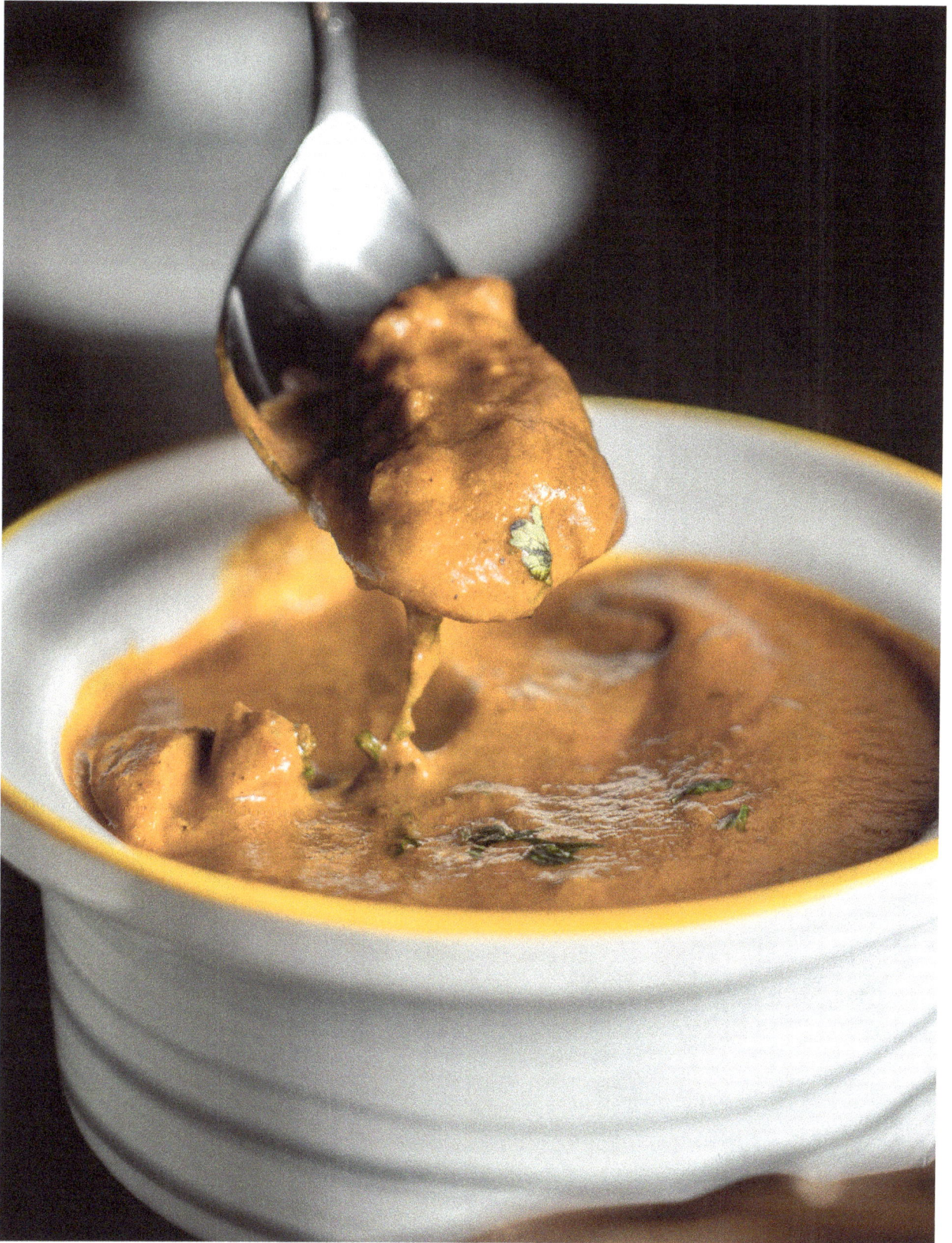

36. Avocado Fries

Ingredients:
- 1 ounce Aquafina
- 1 avocado, sliced
- ½ teaspoon salt
- ½ cup panko breadcrumbs

Air Fryer Required

Preparation time: 10 min.
Cooking time: 15 min.
Servings: 4

Calories: 263
Protein: 7.4g
Fat: 8.2g

Directions:
1. Toss the panko breadcrumbs and salt together in a bowl.
2. Pour Aquafina into another bowl. Dredge the avocado slices in Aquafina and then panko breadcrumbs. Arrange the slices in a single layer in an air fryer basket.
3. Air fry at 390° F for 10 minutes.

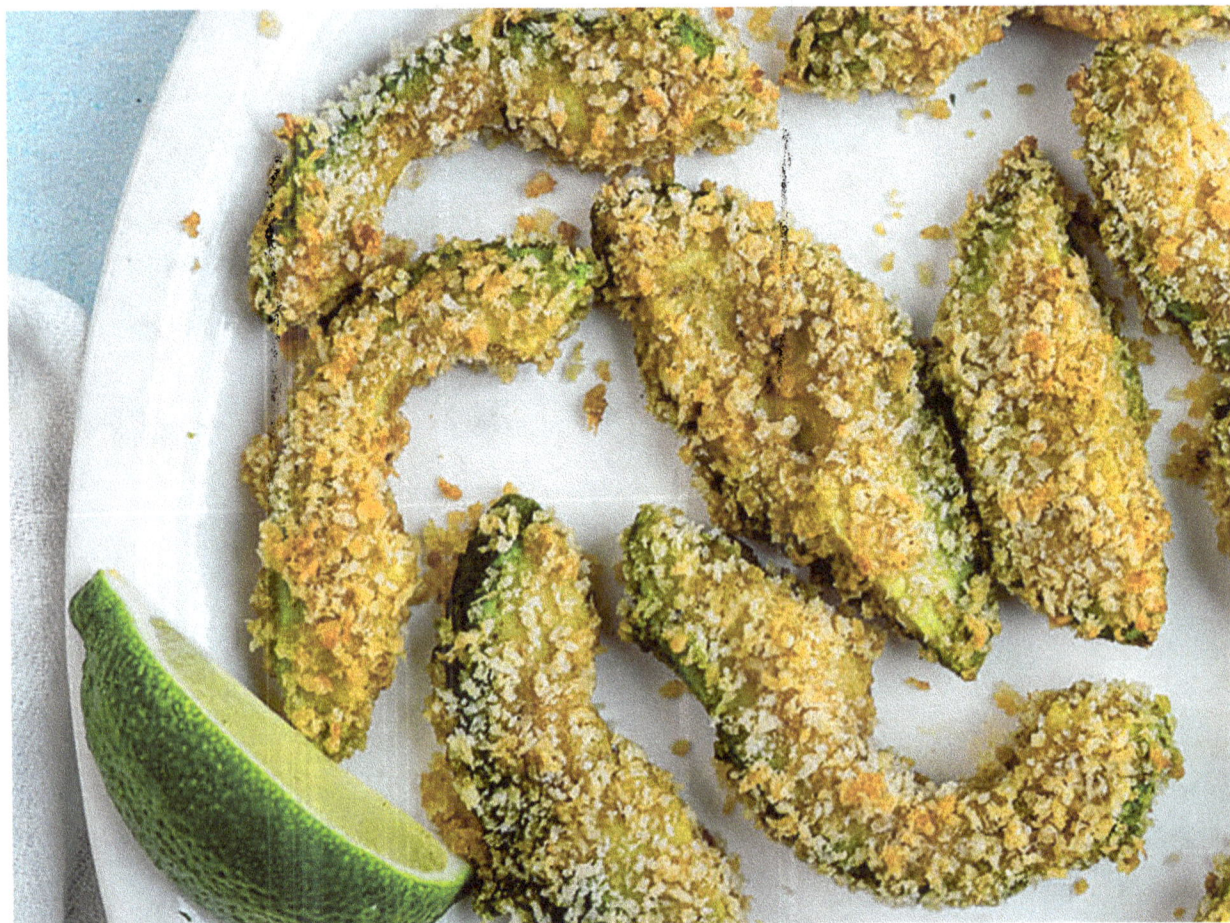

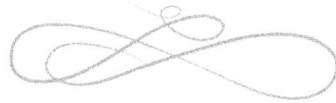

CHAPTER 7

Dinner Recipes

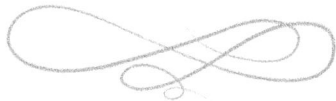

37. Sesame-Crusted Mahi-Mahi

Ingredients:

- 2 tablespoons Dijon mustard
- 1 tablespoon Sour cream, low-fat
- ½ cup Sesame seeds
- 2 tablespoons Olive oil
- 1 Lemon, wedged
- 4 (4 oz. each) Mahi-mahi or sole filets

Preparation time: 5 min.
Cooking time: 13 min.
Servings: 4

Calories: 282
Protein: 18g
Fat: 17g

Directions:

1. Rinse filets and pat dry. In a bowl, mix sour cream and mustard. Spread this mixture on all sides of fish. Roll in sesame seeds to coat.
2. Heat olive oil in a large skillet over medium heat. Pan-fry fish, turning once, for 5–8 minutes or until fish flakes when tested with fork and sesame seeds are toasted. Serve immediately with lemon wedges.

38. Country Chicken

Ingredients:

- ¾ pound Chicken tenders, fresh, boneless skinless
- ½ cup Almond meal
- ½ cup Almond flour
- 1 teaspoon Rosemary, dried
- Salt
- Pepper
- 2 Eggs, beaten

Preparation time: 10 min.
Cooking time: 15 min.
Servings: 2

Calories: 480
Protein: 26g
Fat: 36g

Directions:

1. Rinse the chicken tenders, pat dry.
2. In a medium bowl, pour in almond flour.
3. In a medium bowl, beat the eggs.
4. In a separate bowl, pour in almond meal. Season with rosemary, salt, pepper.
5. Take the chicken pieces and toast in flour, then egg, then almond meal. Set on a tray.
6. Place the tray in the freezer for 5 minutes.
7. Preheat fryer to 350°F. Lightly spray the cook basket with non-stick cooking spray.
8. Cook tenders for 10 minutes. After the timer runs out, set the temperature to 390°F, cook 5 more minutes until golden brown.
9. Serve on a platter. Side with preferred dipping sauce.

39. Cajun Shrimp

Ingredients:

- 16 Tiger shrimp
- 2 tablespoons Cornstarch
- 1 teaspoon Cayenne pepper
- 1 teaspoon Old bay seasoning
- Salt
- Pepper
- 1 teaspoon Olive oil

Preparation time: 10 min.
Cooking time: 5 min.
Servings: 2

Calories: 127
Protein: 7g
Fat: 10g

Directions:

1. Rinse the shrimp. Pat dry.
2. In a bowl, combine corn starch, cayenne pepper, old bay seasoning, salt, pepper. Stir.
3. In a bowl, add the shrimp. Drizzle olive oil over shrimp to lightly coat.
4. Dip the shrimp in seasoning, shake off any excess.
5. Preheat fryer to 375°F. Lightly spray the cook basket with non-stick Keto cooking spray.
6. Transfer to fryer. Cook for 5 minutes; shake after 2 minutes, until cooked thoroughly.
7. Serve on a platter.

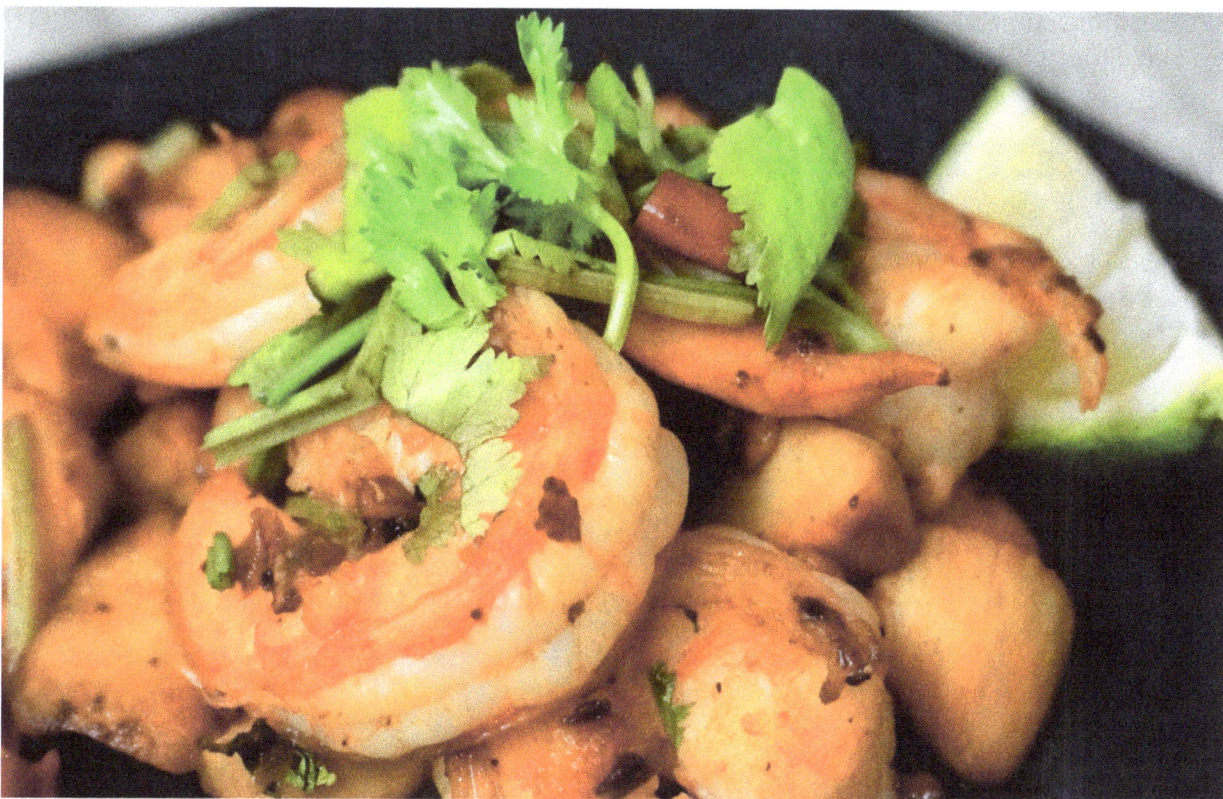

40. Balsamic Chicken with Roasted Vegetables

Ingredients:

- 10 asparaguses, ends trimmed and cut in half
- 8 boneless, skinless chicken thighs, fat trimmed
- 2 bell peppers, sliced into strips
- ½ cup carrots, sliced into half long and cut into 3-inch pieces
- 1 red onion, chopped into large chunks
- ¼ cup + 1 tablespoon balsamic vinegar
- 5 oz. mushrooms, sliced
- 2 tablespoons olive oil
- ½ tablespoon dried oregano
- 2 sage leaves, chopped
- 2 garlic cloves, smashed and chopped
- ½ teaspoon sugar
- 1½ tablespoons rosemary
- 1 teaspoon salt
- Black pepper, to taste
- Cooking spray

Preparation time: 10 min.
Cooking time: 30 min.
Servings: 4

Calories: 450
Protein: 48g
Fat: 17g

Directions:

1. Preheat the oven to 425°F.
2. Season chicken with salt and pepper and spray 2 large baking sheets with cooking spray.
3. Mix all the ingredients in a bowl and mix well. Place everything on the prepared baking sheet and spread it in a single layer.
4. Bake for 25 minutes. Serve.

41. Cheesy Tuna Pesto Pasta

Ingredients:

- 4 cups zucchini noodles, spiralized, cooked
- 1 cup cheddar, grated
- 1 cup yellowfin tuna in olive oil
- 7 oz. basil pesto
- 1½ cup punnet cherry tomato, halved

Preparation time: 10 min.
Cooking time: 25 min.
Servings: 4

Calories: 696
Protein: 40g
Fat: 27g

Directions:

1. Mix pesto and tuna with oil in a bowl. Mash well. Add in 1/3 of the cheese and add all the tomatoes.
2. Add noodles to the bowl, toss well to coat. Transfer the mixture to a baking dish and add the remaining cheese on top.
3. Broil the dish for 4 minutes. Serve.

42. Low Carb Chili

INGREDIENTS:

- 1 bell pepper, chopped
- 1¼ lb. ground beef
- 8 oz. tomato paste
- 1½ tomato, chopped
- 2 celery sticks, chopped
- ½ cup onion, chopped
- 1½ teaspoons cumin
- ¾ cup of water
- 1½ teaspoon chili powder
- 1½ teaspoons salt
- ½ teaspoon pepper

Preparation time: 5 min.
Cooking time: 40 min.
Servings: 6

Calories: 348
Protein: 14.9g
Fat: 28.8g

DIRECTIONS:

1. Cook the meat in a frying pan until brown. Drain the excess fat and season meat with salt.
2. Add peppers and onions to the pan and cook for 2 minutes. Mix onions, cooked meat, peppers, tomatoes, water, celery, and tomato paste in a pot.
3. Add the spices to the pot. Bring to a boil and reduce the heat to low-medium. Cook for 2 hours while stirring every 30 minutes. Serve.

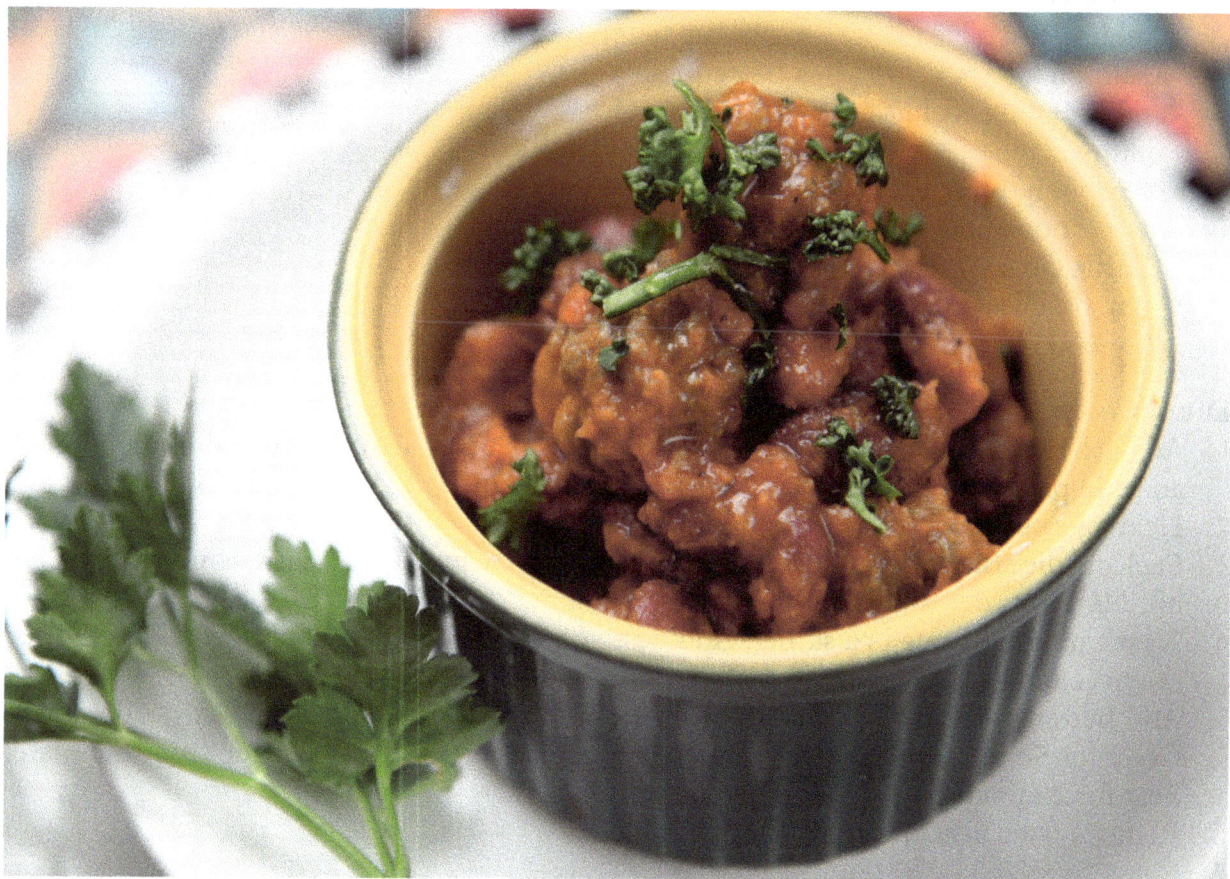

43. KETO MEATLOAF

INGREDIENTS:

- 2 eggs
- 2 lbs. 85% lean grass-fed ground beef
- ¼ cup nutritional yeast
- 1 tablespoon lemon zest
- 2 tablespoons avocado oil
- ¼ cup parsley, chopped
- 4 garlic cloves
- ¼ cup oregano, chopped
- ½ tablespoon pink Himalayan salt
- 1 teaspoon black pepper

Preparation time: 15 min.
Cooking time: 1 hour
Servings: 6

Calories: 344
Protein: 33g
Fat: 29g

DIRECTIONS:

1. Preheat the oven to 400°F. Mix beef, yeast, salt, and pepper in a bowl.
2. Mix eggs, oil, garlic, and herbs in a blender and blend until everything is mixed well. Add this mixture to the beef and mix well.
3. Add the beef mixture to a small loaf pan. Arrange the pan on the middle rack and bake for 1 hour. Remove the pan from the oven. Let cool for 10 minutes. Serve.

44. CRISPY SALMON WITH PESTO CAULIFLOWER RICE

INGREDIENTS:

- 1 tablespoon olive oil
- 3 salmon fillets
- 1 tablespoon coconut aminos
- 1 teaspoon fish sauce
- 1 tablespoon butter
- 3 garlic cloves
- 1 cup basil leaves, chopped
- ¼ cup hemp hearts
- ½ cup olive oil
- 1 lemon juice
- ½ teaspoon pink salt
- 3 cups riced cauliflower, frozen
- 1 scoop MCT Powder
- Pinch salt

Preparation time: 15 min.
Cooking time: 40 min.
Servings: 3

Calories: 647
Protein: 33.8g
Fat: 51g

DIRECTIONS:

1. Add fish sauce, coconut aminos, and olive oil to a baking dish. Pat the salmon fillets dry and add place into the dish skin side down. Add a pinch of salt. Let rest for 20 minutes.
2. Heat an iron skillet on medium heat.
3. Peel and dice the garlic and add it to a blender. Add hemp hearts, basil, lemon juice, olive oil, MCT powder, and salt. Pulse well to combine.
4. Heat cauliflower rice in a skillet. Add pesto and pink salt. Mix well to combine. Lower the heat and keep it warm.
5. Add butter to the iron skillet placed over medium heat. Add salmon skin side down. Cook for 5 minutes. Flip the salmon and add the remaining marinade from the plate. Sear for 2 minutes.
6. Remove from heat and serve on top of rice.
7. Enjoy!

45. ROASTED SHRIMP & BROCCOLI

INGREDIENTS:

- 5 cups broccoli florets
- 1 tablespoon fresh lemon juice
- 1 tablespoon grated lemon rind, divided
- 2 tablespoons extra-virgin olive oil
- Sea salt and pepper, divided
- 1 1/2 pounds large shrimp
- 1/4 teaspoon crushed red pepper

Preparation time: 10 min.
Cooking time: 10 min.
Servings: 4

Calories: 238
Protein: 7.4g
Fat: 35.2g

DIRECTIONS:

1. Preheat the oven to 425°.
2. Add broccoli to boiling water and cook for about 1 minute; transfer to iced water and drain.
3. In a bowl, combine lemon juice, 1½ teaspoons of lemon rind, olive oil, salt and pepper; add shrimp and toss to coat well. Arrange shrimp and broccoli on a greased pan and bake for about 8 minutes or until shrimp is cooked through.
4. In a large bowl, combine the remaining lemon rind, crushed red pepper, salt and pepper; toss in broccoli and serve with shrimp.

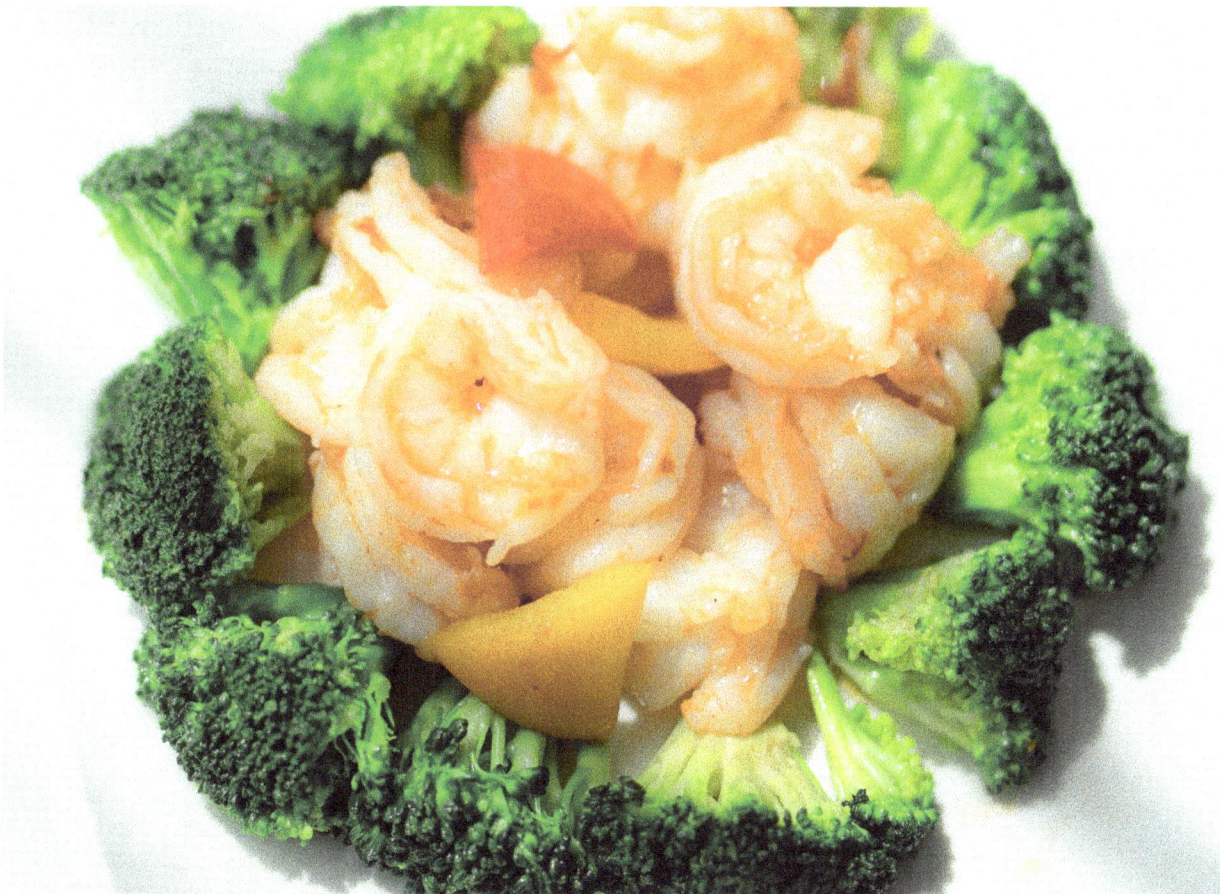

46. PEANUT VEGETABLE PAD THAI

INGREDIENTS:

- 8 ounces brown rice noodles
- 1/3 cup natural peanut butter
- 3 tablespoons unsalted vegetable broth
- 1 tablespoon low-sodium soy sauce
- 2 tablespoons of rice wine vinegar
- 1 tablespoon honey
- 2 teaspoons sesame oil
- 1 teaspoon sriracha (optional)
- 1 tablespoon canola oil
- 1 red bell pepper, thinly sliced
- 1 zucchini, cut into matchsticks
- 2 large carrots, cut into matchsticks
- 3 large eggs, beaten
- ¾ teaspoon kosher or sea salt
- ½ cup unsalted peanuts, chopped
- ½ cup cilantro leaves, chopped

Preparation time: 15 min.
Cooking time: 20 min.
Servings: 6

Calories: 393
Protein: 13g
Fat: 19g

DIRECTIONS:

1. Boil a large pot of water. Cook the rice noodles as stated in package directions. Mix the peanut butter, vegetable broth, soy sauce, rice wine vinegar, honey, sesame oil, and sriracha in a bowl. Set aside.
2. Warm-up canola oil over medium heat in a large nonstick skillet. Add the red bell pepper, zucchini, and carrots, and sauté for 2 to 3 minutes, until slightly soft. Stir in the eggs and fold with a spatula until scrambled. Add the cooked rice noodles, sauce, and salt. Toss to combine. Spoon into bowls and evenly top with the peanuts and cilantro.

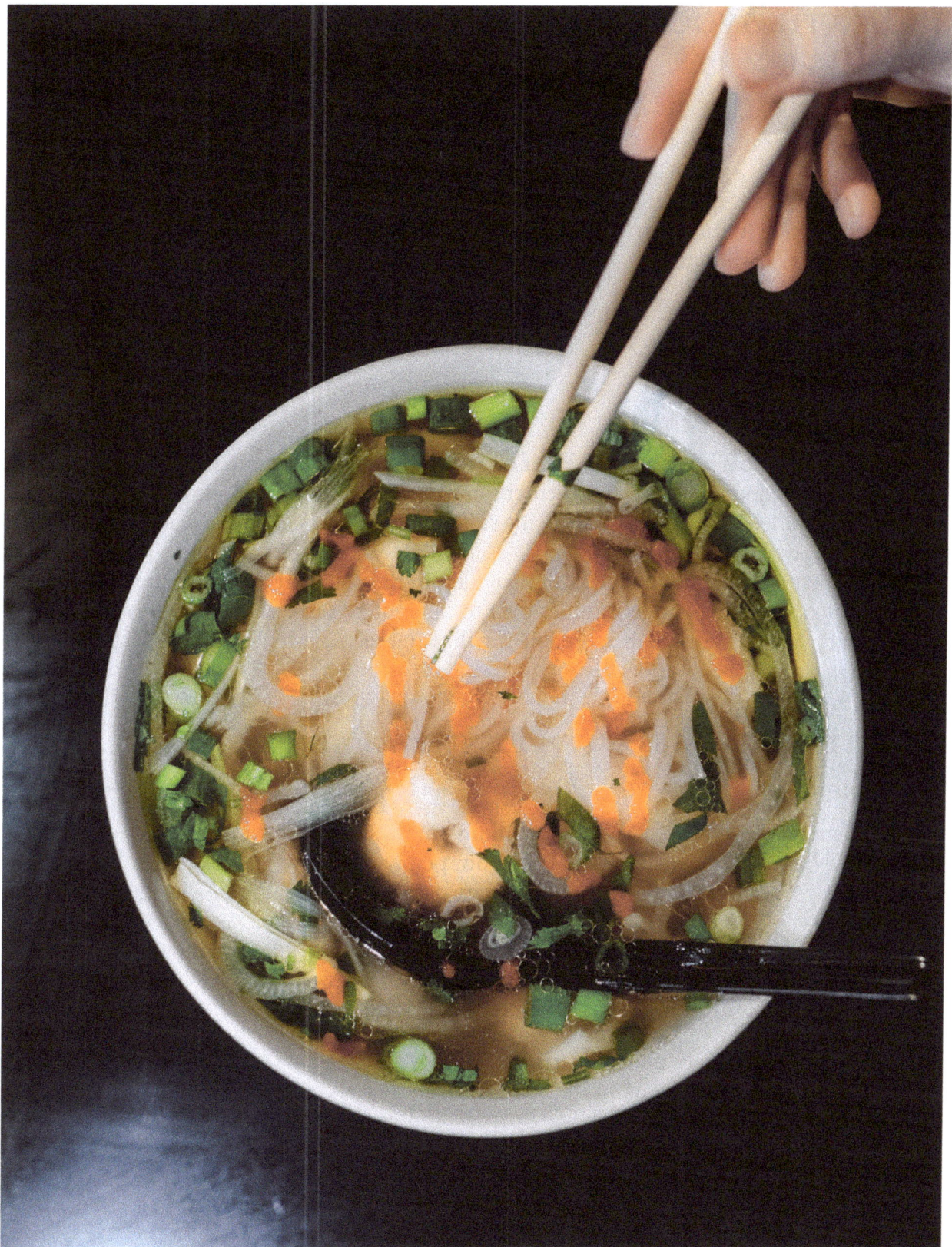

47. LENTIL AVOCADO TACOS

INGREDIENTS:

- 1 tablespoon canola oil
- ½ yellow onion, peeled and diced
- 2-3 garlic cloves, minced
- 1½ cups dried lentils
- ½ teaspoon kosher or sea salt
- 3 to 3½ cups unsalted vegetable or chicken stock
- 2½ tablespoons Taco Seasoning or store-bought low-sodium taco seasoning
- 16 (6-inch) corn tortillas, toasted
- 2 ripe avocados, peeled and sliced

Preparation time: 15 min.
Cooking time: 35 min.
Servings: 6

Calories: 400
Protein: 16g
Fat: 14g

DIRECTIONS:

1. Heat-up the canola oil in a large skillet or Dutch oven over medium heat. Cook the onion within 4 to 5 minutes, until soft. Mix in the garlic and cook within 30 seconds until fragrant. Then add the lentils, salt, and stock. Bring to a simmer for 25 to 35 minutes, adding additional stock if needed.
2. When there's only a small amount of liquid left in the pan, and the lentils are al dente, stir in the taco seasoning and let simmer for 1 to 2 minutes. Taste and adjust the seasoning, if necessary. Spoon the lentil mixture into tortillas and serve with the avocado slices.

48. STEAMED BASS WITH FENNEL, PARSLEY, AND CAPERS

INGREDIENTS:

- 2 5-ounce portions of striped bass
- 2 tablespoons extra-virgin olive oil
- 1/2 lemon, juiced
- 1 fennel bulb, sliced
- 1/4 medium onion, sliced
- 1/4 cup chopped parsley
- 1 tablespoon capers, rinsed
- 1/2 teaspoon sea salt
- Chopped parsley and olive oil, for garnish

Preparation time: 15 min.
Cooking time: 15 min.
Servings: 2

Calories: 325
Protein: 10.9g
Fat: 24.6g

DIRECTIONS:

1. Add lemon juice, fennel and onion to a pan and cover with 1-inch water; bring the mixture to a gentle boil. Lower heat and simmer for about 5 minutes.
2. Add seasoned fish and sprinkle with parsley and capers; cover and simmer for about 10 minutes.
3. Transfer to a serving bowl and drizzle with extra virgin olive oil and top with more parsley to serve.

49. EASY BBQ CHICKEN TOSTADAS

INGREDIENTS:

- 3 cups cooked and shredded chicken
- 2 cups of your favorite barbecue sauce, divided
- 8 tostada shells or 8 corn tortillas brushed lightly with olive oil and baked for 3-5 minutes per side, until crispy

- 3 green onions, very thinly sliced (optional)
- 2 cups shredded cheese (You can choose between mozzarella, cheddar, Monterey Jack, or a blend)

Preparation time: 10 min.
Cooking time: 8 min.
Servings: 4

Calories: 693
Protein: 31g
Fat: 33g

DIRECTIONS:

1. Preheat to 350°F in your oven. Spread out two rimmed baking sheets with the tostada shells (or baked tortillas).
2. In a small bowl, mix the chicken and 1 cup barbecue sauce, and swirl to coat.
3. Divide the chicken between the shells of the tostada and top with the cheese (approximately 1/4 cup each).
4. Bake, only until the cheese is melted, for 6 to 8 minutes.
5. Remove and drizzle with the remaining 1/2 cup of barbecue sauce from the oven. If needed, sprinkle it with green onions.

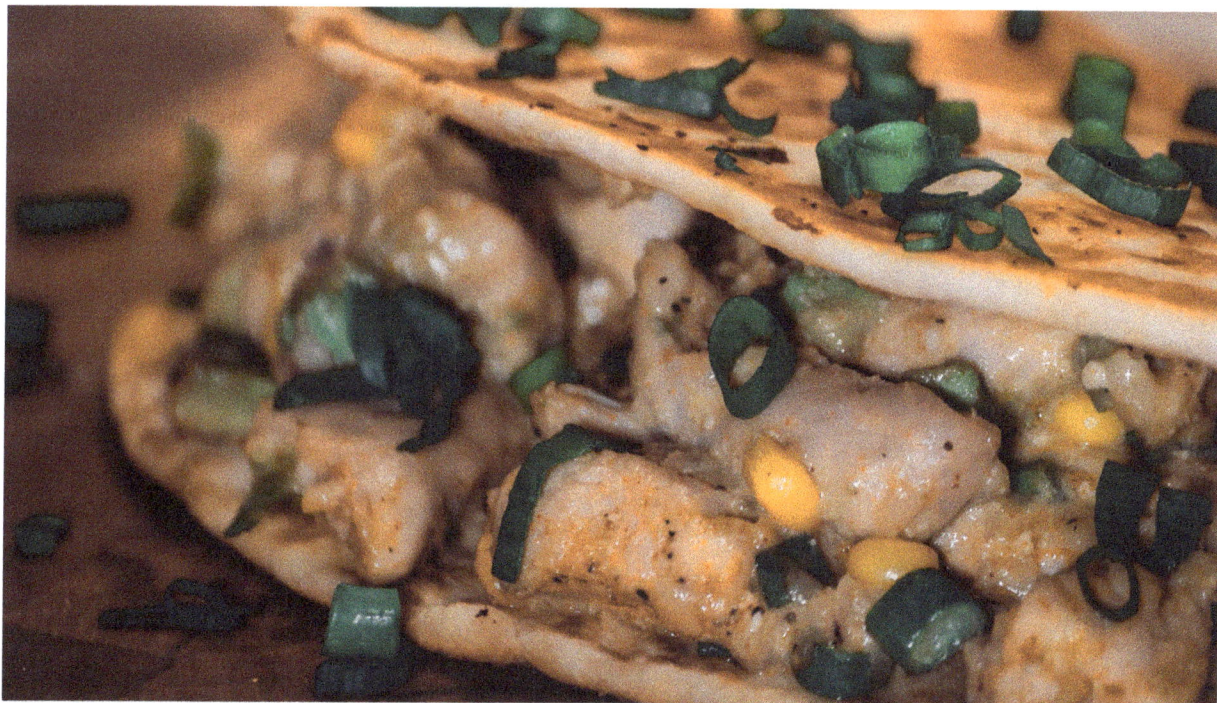

50. Crunchy Chicken w/ Mustard-Orange Vinaigrette Dressing

Ingredients:

Salad

- 1/2 cup chopped cooked chicken
- 1 cup shaved Brussels sprouts
- 2 cups baby spinach
- 2 cups mixed greens
- 1/2 avocado sliced
- Segments of one orange
- 1 teaspoon raw pumpkin seeds
- 1 teaspoon toasted almonds
- 1 teaspoon hemp seeds

Dressing

- 1/2 shallot, chopped
- 1 garlic clove, chopped
- 2 teaspoons balsamic vinegar
- 1 teaspoon extra virgin olive oil
- ½ cup fresh orange juice
- 1 teaspoon Dijon mustard
- 1 teaspoon raw honey
- Fresh ground pepper

Preparation time: 5 min.
Cooking time: 5 min.
Servings: 1

Calories: 365
Protein: 18.8g
Fat: 15.6g

Directions:

1. In a blender, blend together all dressing ingredients until very smooth; set aside.
2. Combine all salad ingredients in a large bowl; drizzle with dressing and toss to coat well before serving.

51. Steamed Salmon w/ Fennel & Fresh Herbs

Ingredients:

- 1 tablespoon extra-virgin olive oil
- 6 ounces wild salmon fillets, skinless
- Fennel fronds
- 1 tablespoon chopped parsley
- 1 tablespoon chopped dill
- 1 tablespoon chopped chives
- 1 tablespoon chopped tarragon
- 1 tablespoon chopped basil
- 1 tablespoon chopped shallot
- 1 tablespoon lemon juice

Preparation time: 15 min.
Cooking time: 6 min.
Servings: 4

Calories: 98
Protein: 8.9g
Fat: 6.3g

Directions:

1. Lightly oil a steamer basket with olive oil; add salmon and fennel wedges and steam for about 6 minutes. In a bowl, combine the chopped herbs, extra virgin olive oil, and shallot and lemon juice; stir until well combined. Season and spoon over cooked fish.

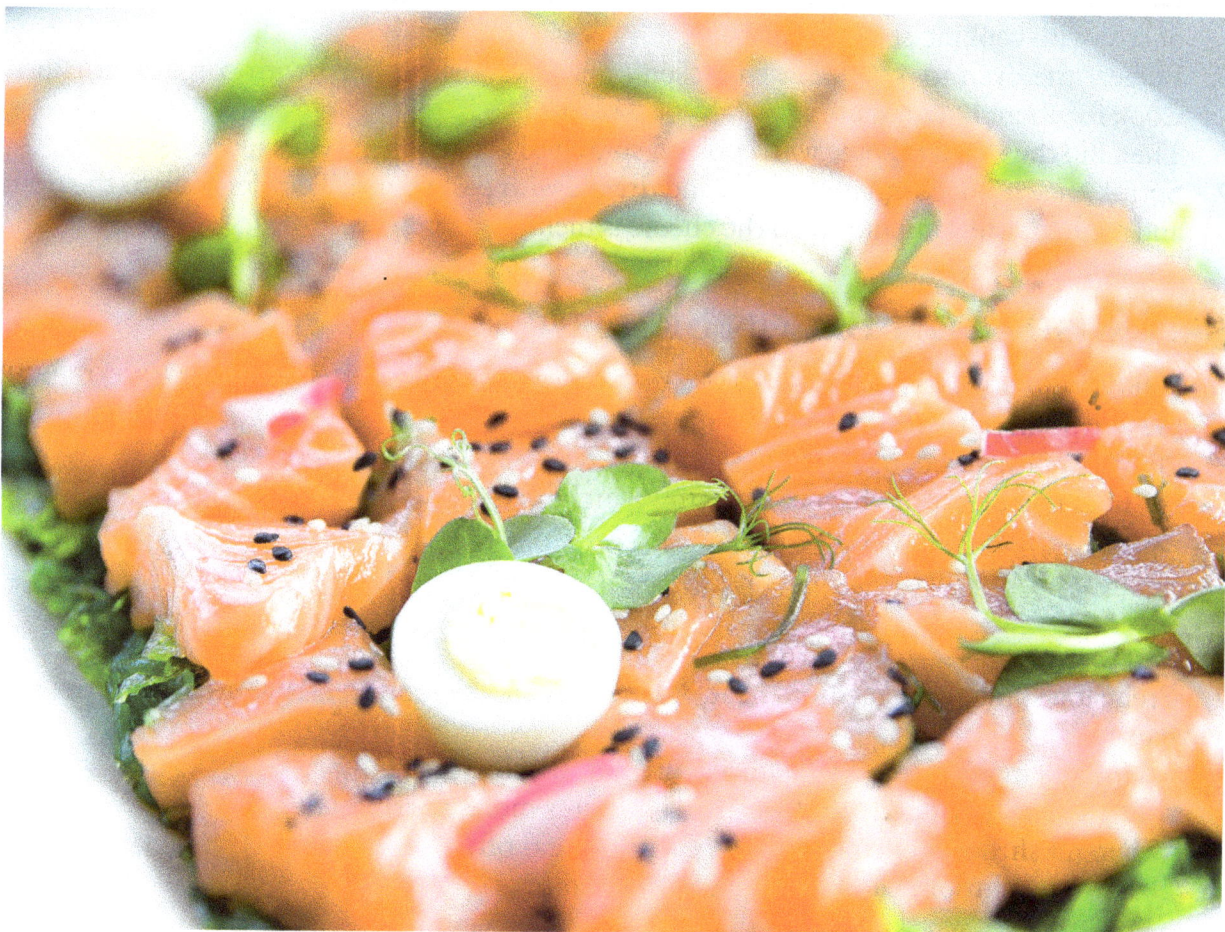

52. CHICKEN PARMESAN

INGREDIENTS:

- 2 lbs. boneless skinless chicken breast
- 4 oz. fresh mozzarella
- 1/3 cup sugar-free marinara
- 1 cup almond flour
- 1 cup parmesan cheese, grated

- 2 eggs
- 1 teaspoon Italian seasoning
- ½ teaspoon black pepper
- ½ teaspoon sea salt

Preparation time: 5 min.
Cooking time: 19 min.
Servings: 8

Calories: 318
Protein: 36g
Fat: 17g

DIRECTIONS:

1. Add chicken to a plastic bag and pound until about ½-inch thick.
2. Add 1 teaspoon Italian seasoning, a cup of parmesan cheese, ½ teaspoon sea salt, a cup of almond flour, and ½ teaspoon pepper. Mix well.
3. Add eggs to a separate bowl and whisk well. Pat dry the chicken with paper towels.
4. Dip chicken into the egg mixture and then coat with almond flour mixture. Brush with oil or coat with cooking spray.
5. Preheat the oven to 425°F. Place chicken on a baking sheet lined with parchment paper. Cook for about 11-12 minutes.
6. Then flip the chicken, spray with cooking spray and cook for 5 minutes more.
7. Sprinkle each piece with mozzarella and drizzle with pasta sauce. Transfer back to the oven and cook for a few minutes until the cheese is melted.

53. MUSHROOM BACON SKILLET

INGREDIENTS:

- ½ teaspoon salt
- 1 tablespoon garlic, minced
- 4 slices pastured pork bacon, cut into ½-inch pieces
- 2 sprigs thyme, leaves only
- 2 cups mushrooms, halved

Preparation time: 5 min.
Cooking time: 10 min.
Servings: 1

Calories: 313
Protein: 13.6g
Fat: 8.5g

DIRECTIONS:

1. Preheat a skillet over medium heat. Add bacon and cook until crispy. Remove from the pan.
2. Add sliced mushrooms. Sauté until softened, stirring often.
3. Add garlic, thyme, and salt. Cook for 5 minutes more, stirring often.
4. When mushrooms become golden, turn the heat off.
5. Garnish mushroom bacon with greens and enjoy!

54. VEGGIE & BEEF SALAD BOWL

INGREDIENTS:

- 2 tablespoons dry red quinoa
- 1/2 cup chopped broccoli florets
- 3 ounces cooked lean beef, diced
- 2 cups mixed greens (arugula, baby spinach, romaine lettuce)
- 1/4 red bell pepper, chopped
- 1 teaspoon red wine vinegar
- 2 teaspoons extra virgin olive oil

Preparation time: 10 min.
Cooking time: 15 min.
Servings: 2

Calories: 145
Protein: 4.2g
Fat: 10.2g

DIRECTIONS:

1. Follow package directions to cook quinoa.
2. In a large bowl, toss cooked quinoa with broccoli, beef, greens, and bell pepper.
3. In a small bowl, whisk together vinegar and oil and pour over the salad. Serve.

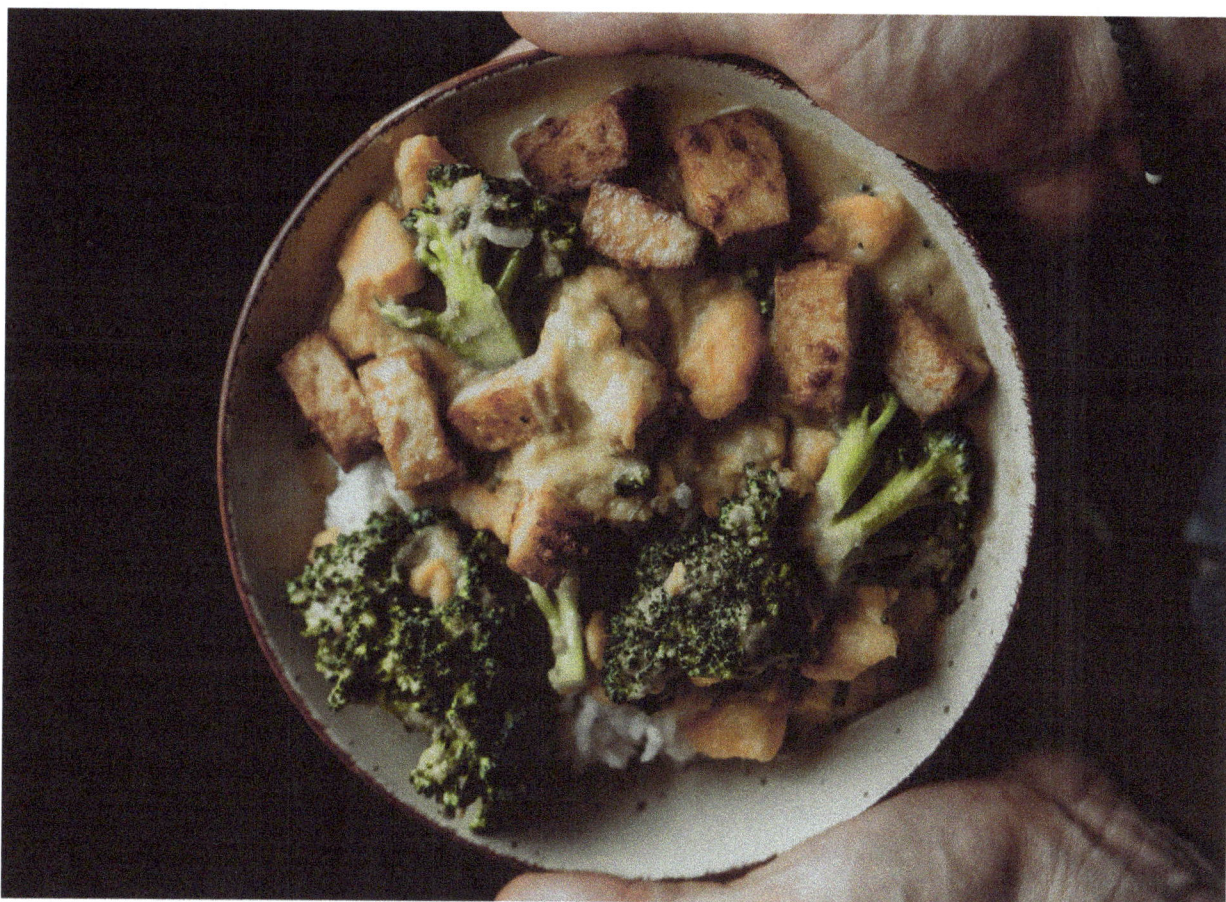

55. LEMON GARLIC SALMON

INGREDIENTS:

- 1 teaspoon extra virgin olive oil
- 4 salmon fillets
- 3 tablespoons freshly squeezed lemon juice
- 1 tablespoon coconut milk
- 1 teaspoon ground pepper
- 1 teaspoon dried parsley flakes
- 1 finely chopped clove garlic

Preparation time: 15 min.
Cooking time: 30 min.
Servings: 4

Calories: 248
Protein: 34.8g
Fat: 12g

DIRECTIONS:

1. Preheat your oven to 190°C (275°F). Coat a baking dish with extra virgin olive oil.
2. Rinse the fish under water and pat dry with paper towels.
3. Arrange the fish fillet in the coated baking dish and drizzle with lemon juice and coconut oil. Sprinkle with ground pepper, parsley and garlic.
4. Bake in the oven for about 30 minutes or until the flakes easily when touched with a fork.

56. TERIYAKI FISH W/ ZUCCHINI

INGREDIENTS:

- 2 (6-ounce) salmon fillets
- 7 tablespoons teriyaki sauce (low-sodium)
- 2 tablespoons sesame seeds
- 2 teaspoons canola oil
- 4 scallions, chopped
- 2 small zucchini, thinly sliced

Preparation time: 10 min.
Cooking time: 10 hours
Servings: 2

Calories: 408
Protein: 40.3g
Fat: 19.9g

DIRECTIONS:

1. Mix fish with 5 tablespoons of teriyaki sauce in a zip-top bag and marinate for at least 20 minutes.
2. In a skillet set over medium heat, toast sesame seeds; set aside. Drain the marinated fish and discard the marinade.
3. Add fish to the skillet and cook for about 5 minutes; remove fish from skillet and keep warm.
4. Add oil, scallions and zucchini to the skillet and sauté for about 4 minutes or until browned.
5. Stir in the remaining teriyaki sauce and sprinkle with toasted sesame seeds; serve with fish.

57. Baked Salmon with Dill-Avocado Yogurt

Ingredients:

- 1/2 cup Greek yogurt
- 1 avocado, diced
- 2 tablespoons lemon juice
- 1 clove garlic
- 3 tablespoons chopped dill
- 4 (6-ounce) salmon fillets
- 1 tablespoon extra-virgin olive oil
- Pinch of sea salt
- Pinch of black pepper

Preparation time: 10 min.
Cooking time: 10 min.
Servings: 4

Calories: 388
Protein: 24.5g
Fat: 1.6g

Directions:

1. Preheat the oven to 400°F.
2. In a blender, blend together Greek yogurt, avocado, 1 tablespoon water, lemon juice, garlic, dill, salt and pepper until very smooth; set aside.
3. Place salmon skin side down onto a foil lined baking sheet and drizzle with extra virgin olive oil; season with salt and pepper and bake for about 10 minutes or until cooked through. Serve salmon topped with dill-avocado yogurt.

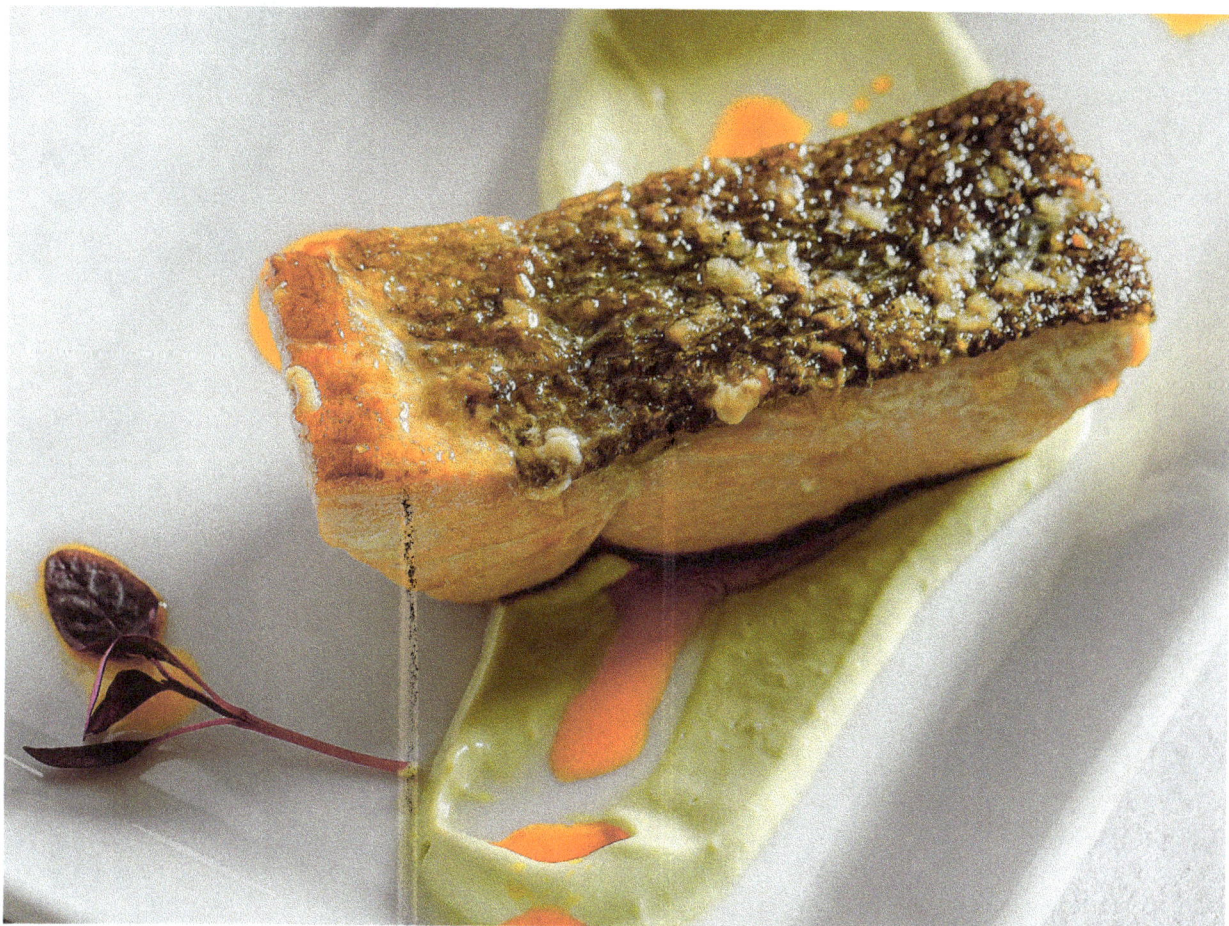

58. Crockpot Coconut Curry Shrimp

INGREDIENTS:

- 1 pound shrimp, with shells
- 15 ounces water
- 30 ounces light coconut milk
- ½ cup Thai red curry sauce
- ¼ cup cilantro
- 2½ teaspoon lemon garlic seasoning

Preparation time: 5 min.
Cooking time: 2 hours
Servings: 8

Calories: 312
Protein: 15.3g
Fat: 26.3g

DIRECTIONS:

1. In a slow cooker, combine water, coconut milk, red curry paste, cilantro, and lemon garlic seasoning; stir to mix well and cook on high for about 2 hours. Add shrimp and continue cooking for another 30 minutes or until shrimp is cooked through.
2. Serve garnished with cilantro.

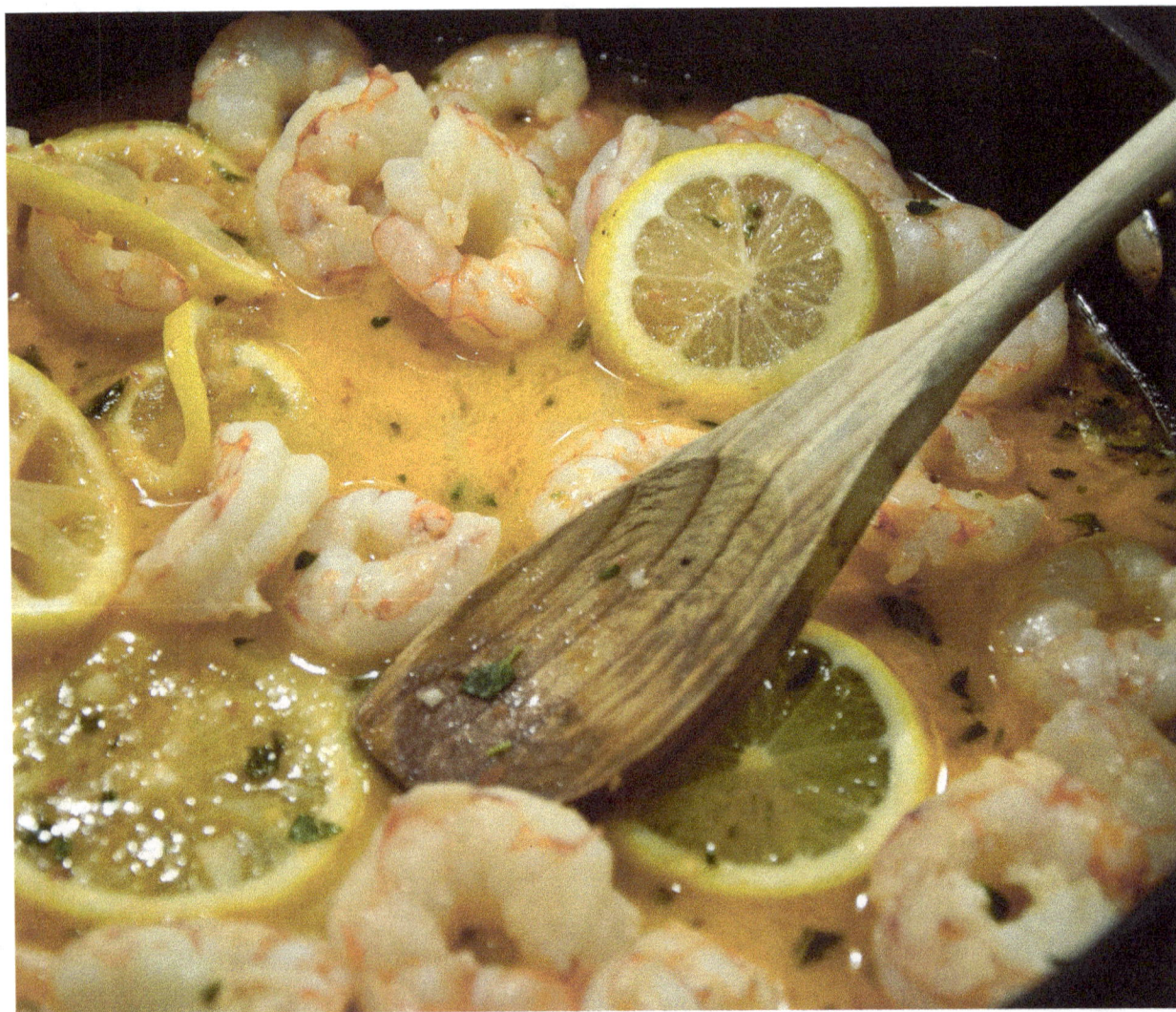

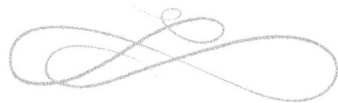

CHAPTER 8

Quick & Easy
Recipes

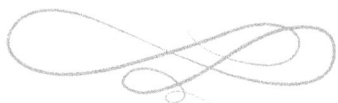

59. ROASTED BRUSSELS SPROUTS WITH PECANS AND GORGONZOLA

INGREDIENTS:

- 1 pound Brussels Sprouts, fresh
- ¼ cup Pecans, chopped
- 1 tablespoon Olive oil
- Extra olive oil to oil the baking tray
- Pepper and salt for tasting
- ¼ cup Gorgonzola cheese (If you prefer not to use the Gorgonzola cheese, you can toss the Brussels sprouts when hot, with 2 tablespoons of butter instead.

Preparation time: 10 min.
Cooking time: 35 min.
Servings: 4

Calories: 149
Protein: 5g
Fat: 11g

DIRECTIONS:

1. Warm the oven to 350 degrees Fahrenheit or 175 Celsius.
2. Rub a large pan or any vessel you wish to use with a little bit of olive oil. You can use a paper towel or a pastry brush.
3. Cut off the ends of the Brussels sprouts if you need to and then cut then in a lengthwise direction into halves. (Fear not if a few of the leaves come off of them, some may become deliciously crunchy during cooking)
4. Chop up all of the pecans using a knife and then measure them for the amount.
5. Put your Brussels sprouts as well as the sliced pecans inside a bowl, and cover them all with some olive oil, pepper, and salt (be generous).
6. Arrange all of your pecans and Brussels sprouts onto your roasting pan in a single layer
7. Roast this for 30 to 35 minutes, or when they become tender and can be pierced with a fork easily. Stir during cooking if you wish to get a more even browning.
8. Once cooked, toss them with the Gorgonzola Cheese (or butter) before you serve them. Serve them hot.

60. STUFFED BEEF LOIN IN STICKY SAUCE

INGREDIENTS:

- 1 tablespoon Erythritol
- 1 tablespoon lemon juice
- 4 tablespoons water
- 1 tablespoon butter
- ½ teaspoon tomato sauce
- ¼ teaspoon dried rosemary
- 9 ounces beef loin
- 3 ounces celery root, grated
- 3 ounces bacon, sliced
- 1 tablespoon walnuts, chopped
- ¾ teaspoon garlic, diced
- 2 teaspoons butter
- 1 tablespoon olive oil
- 1 teaspoon salt
- ½ cup of water

Preparation time: 15 min.
Cooking time: 6 min.
Servings: 4

Calories: 321
Protein: 18.35g
Fat: 26.68g

DIRECTIONS:

1. Cut the beef loin into the layer and spread it with the dried rosemary, butter, and salt. Then place over the beef loin: grated celery root, sliced bacon, walnuts, and diced garlic.
2. Roll the beef loin and brush it with olive oil. Secure the meat with the help of the toothpicks. Place it in the tray and add a ½ cup of water.
3. Cook the meat in the preheated to 365F oven for 40 minutes.
4. Meanwhile, make the sticky sauce:
5. Mix up together Erythritol, lemon juice, 4 tablespoons of water, and butter.
6. Preheat the mixture until it starts to boil. Then add tomato sauce and whisk it well.
7. Bring the sauce to boil and remove from the heat.
8. When the beef loin is cooked, remove it from the oven and brush with the cooked sticky sauce very generously.
9. Slice the beef roll and sprinkle with the remaining sauce.

61. Roasted Broccoli

Ingredients:

- 4 cups broccoli florets
- 1 tablespoon olive oil
- Salt and pepper to taste

Preparation time: 5 min.
Cooking time: 20 mins
Servings: 4

Calories: 62
Protein: 4g
Fat: 4g

Directions:

1. Preheat your oven to 400 degrees F
2. Add broccoli in a zip bag alongside oil and shake until coated
3. Add seasoning and shake again
4. Spread broccoli out on the baking sheet, bake for 20 minutes
5. Let it cool and serve.

62. Squash Bites

Ingredients:

- 10 ounces of turkey meat, cooked, sliced
- 2 pounds butternut squash, cubed
- 1 teaspoon chili powder
- 1 teaspoon garlic powder
- 1 teaspoon sweet paprika
- Black pepper to taste

Preparation time: 10 min.
Cooking time: 40 mins
Servings: 4

Calories: 223
Protein: 23g
Fat: 3.8g

Directions:

1. In a bowl, mix butternut squash cubes with chili powder, black pepper, garlic powder and paprika and toss to coat.
2. Wrap squash pieces in turkey slices, place them all on a lined baking sheet, place in the oven at 350 degrees F, bake for 20 minutes, flip and bake for 20 minutes more.
3. Arrange squash bites on a platter and serve. Enjoy

63. Parmesan Crisps

Ingredients:
- 1 teaspoon butter
- 8 ounces parmesan cheese, full fat and shredded

Preparation time: 5 min.
Cooking time: 25 mins
Servings: 8

Calories: 133
Protein: 11g
Fat: 11g

Directions:
1. Preheat your oven to 400 degrees F
2. Put parchment paper on a baking sheet and grease with butter
3. Spoon parmesan into 8 mounds, spreading them apart evenly
4. Flatten them
5. Bake for 5 minutes until browned
6. Let them cool
7. Serve and enjoy.

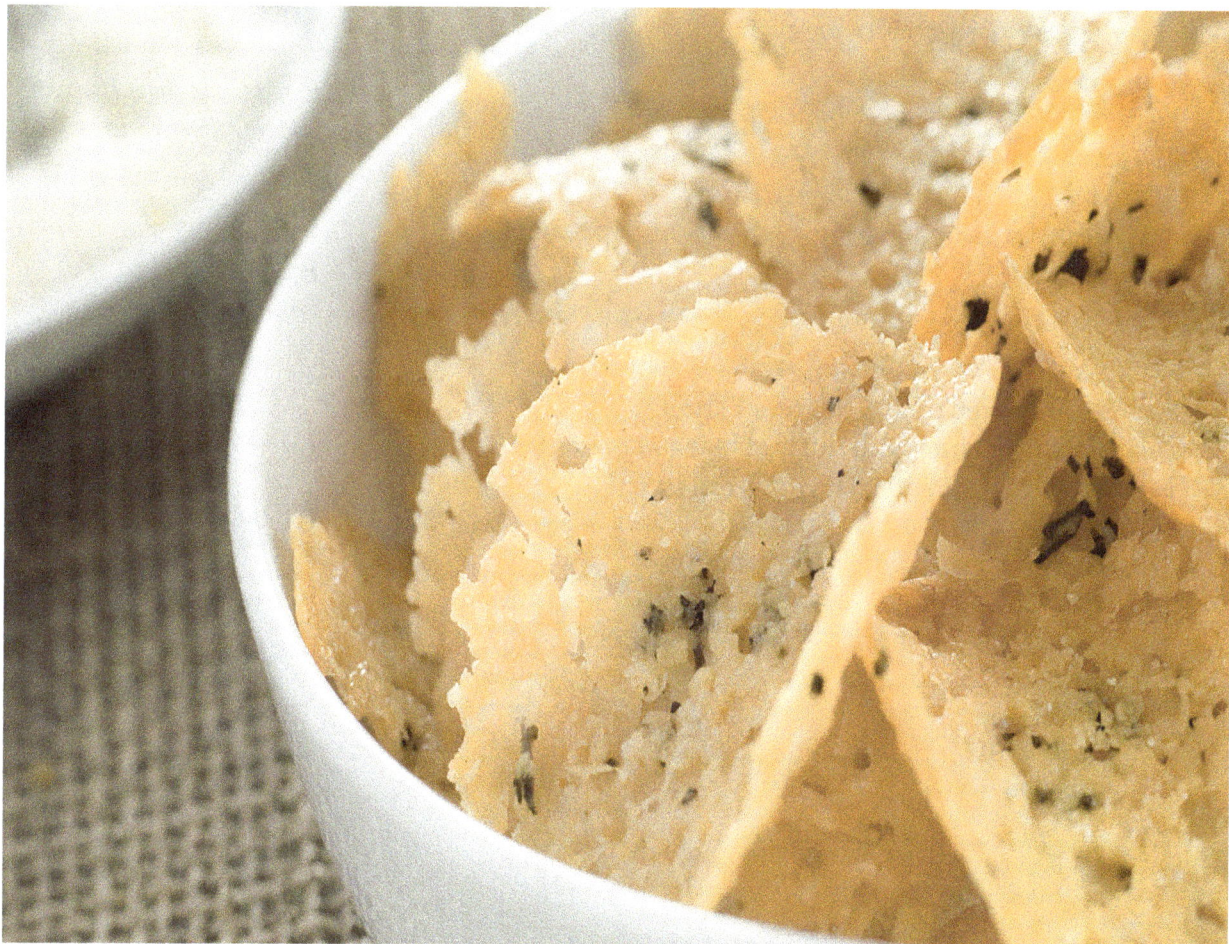

64. ARTICHOKE PETALS BITES

INGREDIENTS:

- 8 ounces artichoke petals, boiled, drained, without salt
- ½ cup almond flour
- 4 ounces Parmesan, grated
- 2 tablespoons almond butter, melted

Preparation time: 10 min.
Cooking time: 10 min.
Servings: 8

Calories: 93
Protein: 6.54g
Fat: 3.72g

DIRECTIONS:
1. In the mixing bowl, mix up together almond flour and grated Parmesan.
2. Preheat the oven to 355F.
3. Dip the artichoke petals in the almond butter and then coat in the almond flour mixture.
4. Place them in the tray.
5. Transfer the tray in the preheated oven and cook the petals for 10 minutes.
6. Chill the cooked petal bites little before serving.

65. EGGPLANT FRIES

INGREDIENTS:

- 2 eggs
- 2 cups almond flour
- 2 tablespoons coconut oil, spray
- 2 eggplant, peeled and cut thinly
- Salt and pepper

Preparation time: 10 min.
Cooking time: 15 min.
Servings: 8

Calories: 212
Protein: 8.6g
Fat: 15.8g

DIRECTIONS:
1. Preheat your oven to 400 degrees Fahrenheit
2. Take a bowl and mix with salt and black pepper in it
3. Take another bowl and beat eggs until frothy
4. Dip the eggplant pieces into eggs
5. Then coat them with flour mixture
6. Add another layer of flour and egg
7. Then, take a baking sheet and grease with coconut oil on top
8. Bake for about 15 minutes
9. Serve and enjoy.

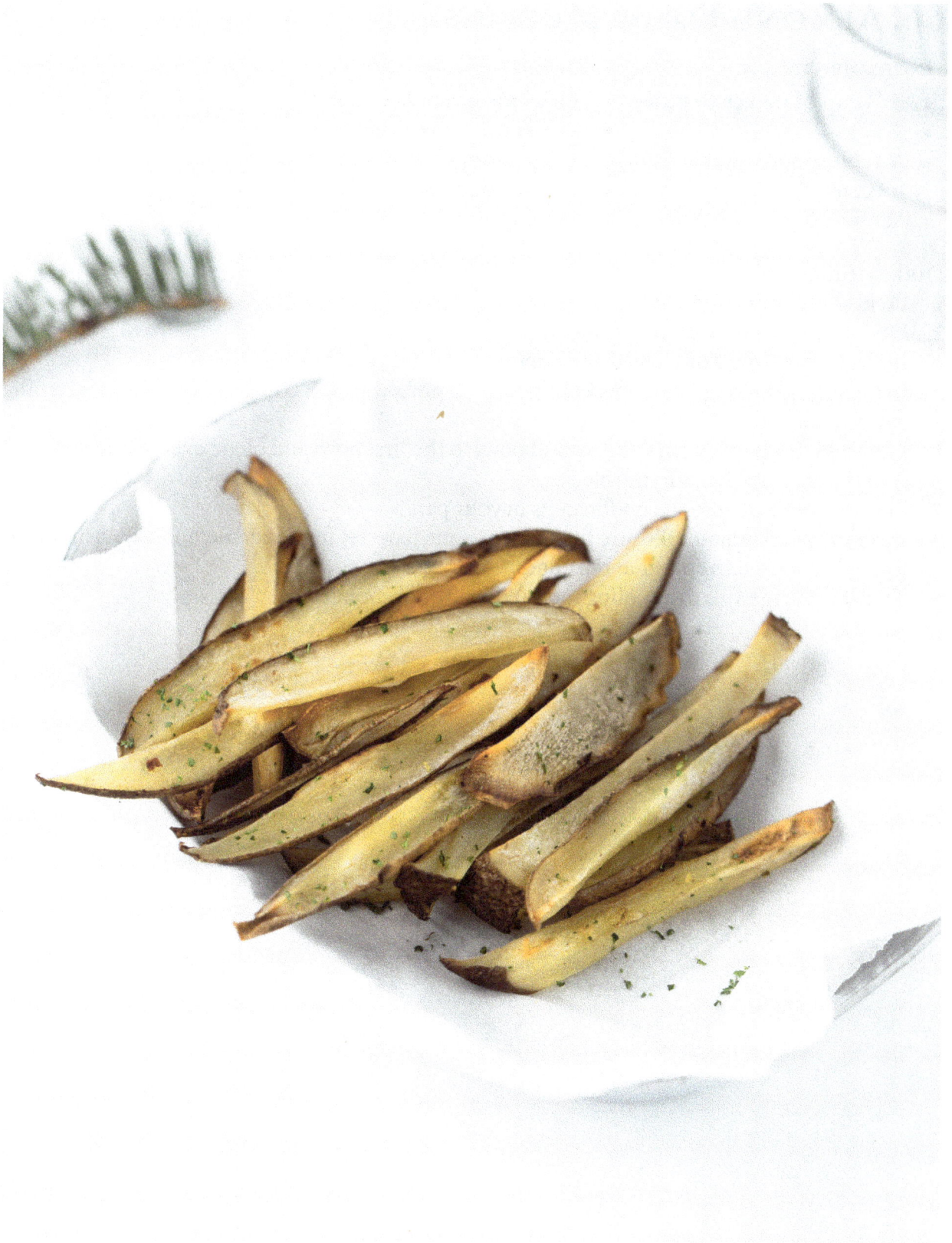

66. ALMOND FLOUR MUFFINS

INGREDIENTS:

- 1/3 cup of pumpkin puree
- 3 eggs
- 2 tablespoons agave nectar
- 2 tablespoons coconut oil
- 1 teaspoon vanilla extract
- 1 teaspoon white vinegar
- 1 cup chopped fruits
- 1 teaspoon baking soda
- ½ teaspoon salt

Preparation time: 15 min.
Cooking time: 30 mins
Servings: 8

Calories: 75
Protein: 0g
Fat: 6g

DIRECTIONS:

1. Preheat the oven to 350°F.
2. Line the muffin tin with paper liners
3. In the first mixing bowl, whisk the almond flour, salt, and baking soda.
4. In the second mixing bowl, whisk the pumpkin puree, eggs, coconut oil, agave nectar, vanilla extract, and vinegar.
5. Now add this puree mix of the second bowl to the first bowl and blend everything well.
6. Add the chopped fruits to the blend.
7. Pour the mixture into the muffin cups in your pan.
8. Bake for 15-20 minutes. Ensure that the contents have set in the center, and a golden brown lining has started to appear at the edges.
9. Transfer the muffins to a cooling rack and let it cool completely.

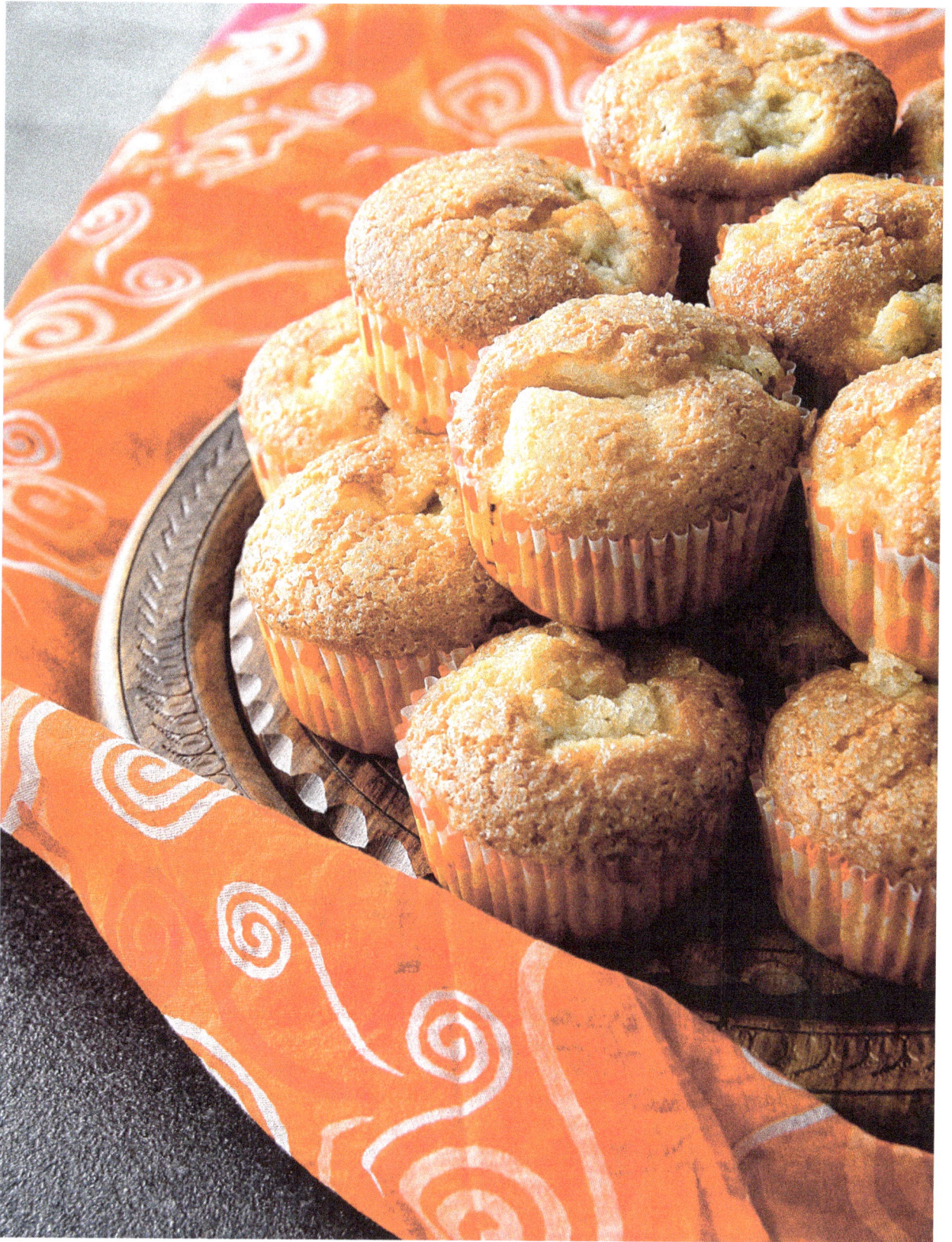

67. Zucchini Chips

Ingredients:

- 1 zucchini, thinly sliced
- A pinch of sea salt
- Black pepper to taste
- 1 teaspoon thyme, dried
- 1 egg
- 1 teaspoon garlic powder
- 1 cup almond flour

Preparation time: 10 min.
Cooking time: 12 min.
Servings: 4

Calories: 106
Protein: 5.1g
Fat: 8.2g

Directions:

1. In a bowl, whisk the egg with a pinch of salt.
2. Put the flour in another bowl and mix it with thyme, black pepper, and garlic powder.
3. Dredge zucchini slices in the egg mix and then in flour.
4. Arrange chips on a lined baking sheet, place in the oven at 450 degrees F and bake for 6 minutes on each side,
5. Serve the zucchini chips as a snack. Enjoy.

68. Very Berry Antioxidant Smoothie

Ingredients:

- 1 banana
- 1¼ cups unsweetened plant-based milk
- ½ cup frozen strawberries
- ½ cup frozen blueberries
- ½ cup frozen raspberries
- 3 pitted Medjool dates
- 1 tablespoon hulled hemp seeds
- ½ tablespoon ground flaxseed
- 1 teaspoon ground chia seeds

Preparation time: 5 min.
Cooking time: 0 min.
Servings: 1

Calories: 538
Protein: 10g
Fat: 11g

Directions:

1. In a blender, combine all the ingredients and blend until smooth.
2. Serve immediately or store in the freezer in a resalable jar.

69. PEPPERONI BITES

INGREDIENTS:

- 1/3 cup tomatoes, chopped
- ½ cup bell peppers, mixed and chopped
- 24 pepperoni slices
- ½ cup tomato sauce
- 4 ounces almond cheese, cubed
- 2 tablespoons basil, chopped
- Black pepper to taste

Preparation time: 5 min.
Cooking time: 10 min.
Servings: 24 pieces

Calories: 59
Protein: 2.5g
Fat: 4.5g

DIRECTIONS:

1. Divide pepperoni slices into a muffin tray.
2. Divide tomato and bell pepper pieces into the pepperoni cups.
3. Also divide the tomato sauce, basil and almond cheese cubes, sprinkle black pepper at the end, place cups in the oven at 400 degrees F and bake for 10 minutes.
4. Arrange the pepperoni bites on a platter and serve.

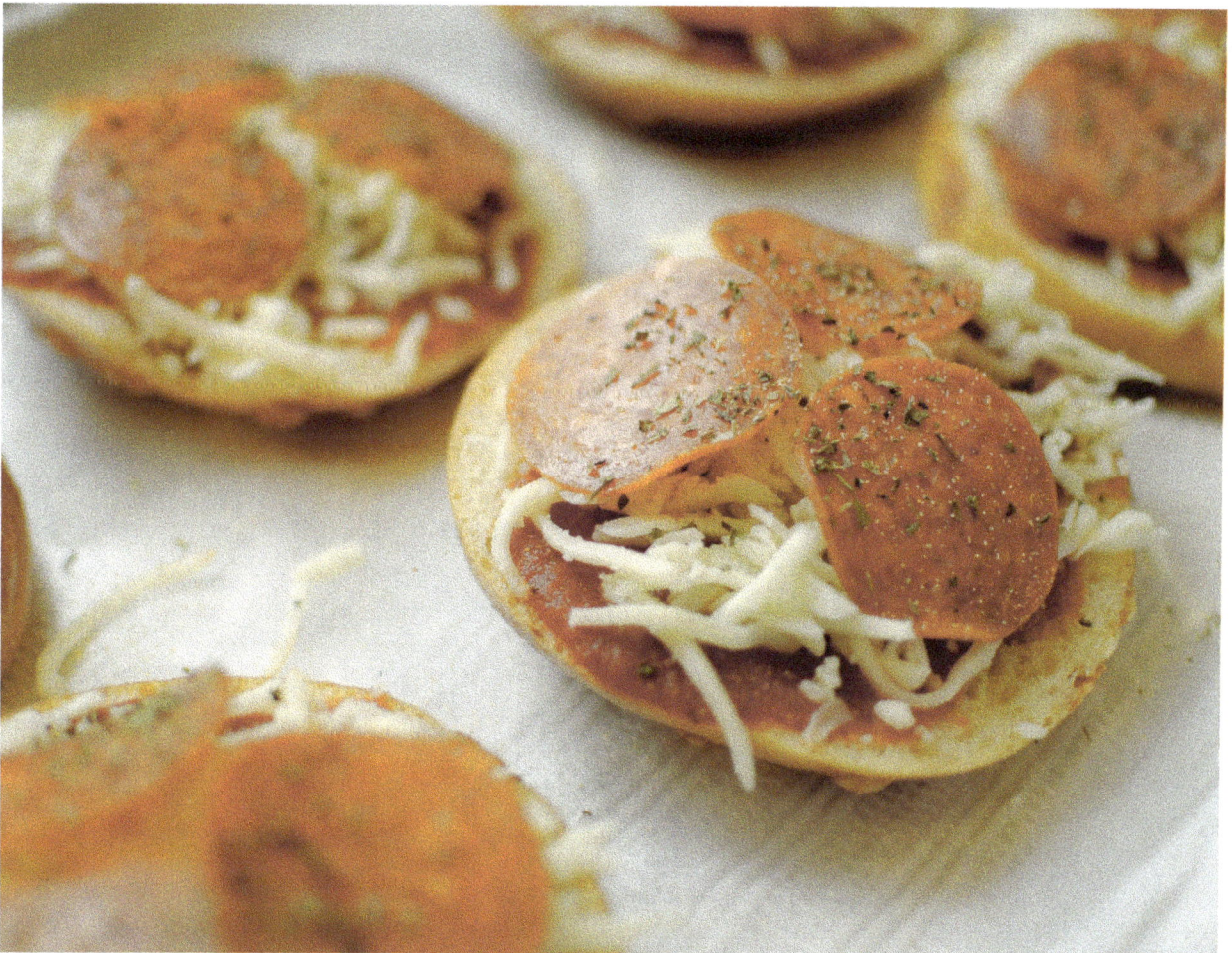

70. GREEN POWER SMOOTHIE

INGREDIENTS:

- 3 cups fresh spinach
- 1½ cups frozen pineapple
- 1 cup unsweetened plant-based milk
- 1 cup fresh kale
- 1 Granny Smith apple, peeled, cored, and chopped
- ½ small avocado, pitted and peeled
- ½ teaspoon spirulina
- 1 tablespoon hemp seeds and peeled
- ½ teaspoon spirulina
- 1 tablespoon hemp seeds

Preparation time: 5 min.
Cooking time: 0 min.
Servings: 1

Calories: 431
Protein: 13g
Fat: 16g

DIRECTIONS:

1. In a blender, combine all the ingredients and blend until smooth.
2. Serve immediately or store in the freezer in a resalable jar.

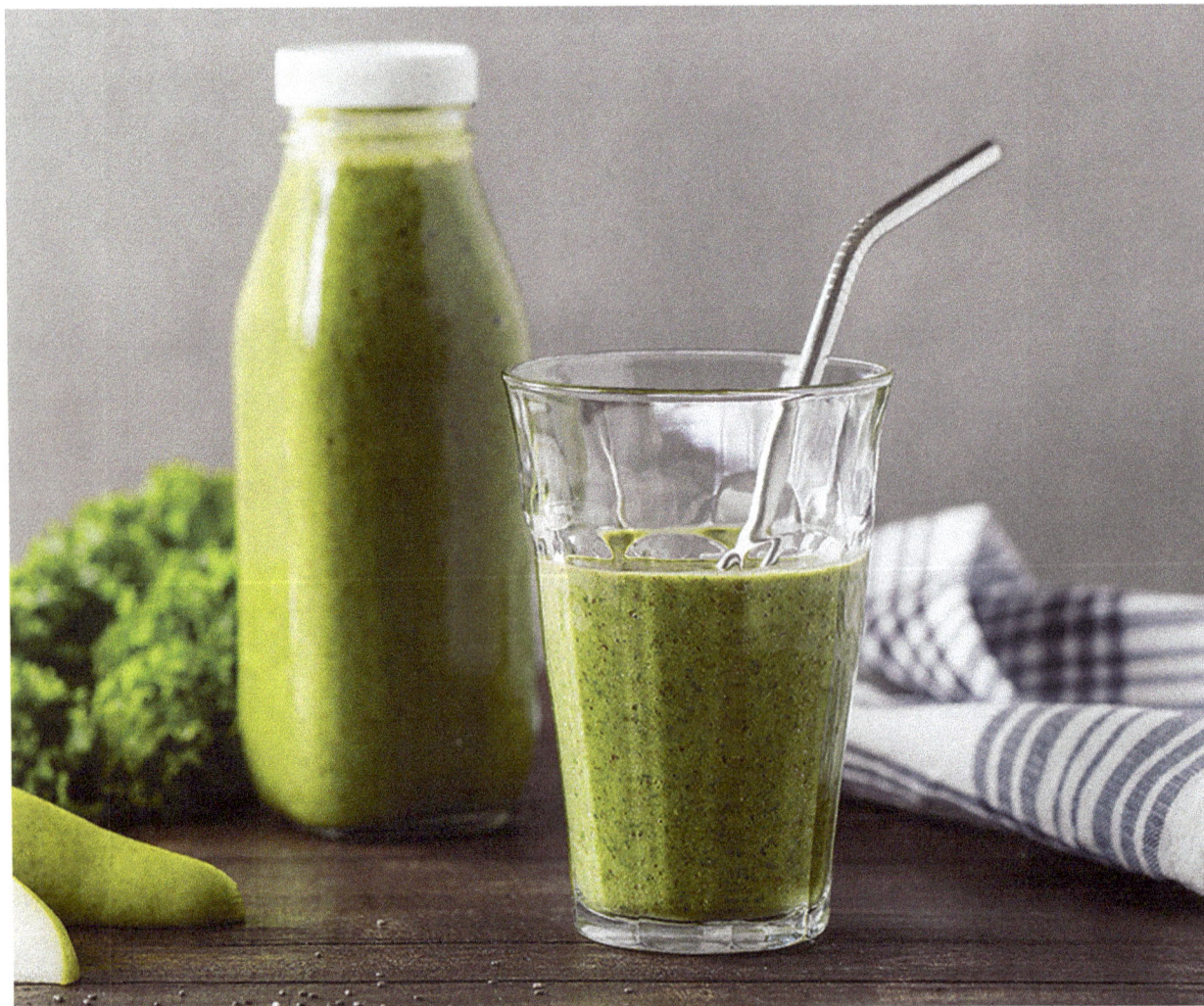

Cooking Conversion

WEIGHT COVERSION	
½ oz.	15g
1 oz.	30g
2 oz.	60g
3 oz.	85g
4 oz.	110g
5 oz.	140g
6 oz.	170g
7 oz.	200g
8 oz.	225g
9 oz.	255g
10 oz.	280g
11 oz.	310g
12 oz.	340g
13 oz.	370g
14 oz.	400g
15 oz.	425g
1 lb.	450g

LIQUID VOLUME MEASUREMENTS

TABLESPOONS	TEASPOONS	FLUID OUNCES	CUPS
16	48	8 fl. Oz.	1
12	36	6 fl. Oz.	¾
8	24	4 fl. Oz.	½
5 ½	16	2 2/3 fl. Oz.	1/3
4	12	2 fl. Oz.	¼
1	3	0.5 fl. Oz.	1/16

LIQUID VOLUME CONVERSION

CUPS / TABLESPOONS	FL. OUNCES	MILLILITERS
1 cup	8 fl. Oz.	240 ml
¾ cup	6 fl. Oz.	180 ml
2/3 cup	5 fl. Oz.	150 ml
½ cup	4 fl. Oz.	120 ml
1/3 cup	2 ½ fl. Oz.	75 ml
¼ cup	2 fl. Oz.	60 ml
1/8 cup	1 fl. Oz.	30 ml
1 tablespoon	½ fl. Oz.	15 ml

TEASPOON (tsp.) / TABLESPOON (Tbsp.)	MILLILITERS
1 tsp.	5ml
2 tsp.	10ml
1 Tbsp.	15ml
2 Tbsp.	30ml
3 Tbsp.	45ml
4 Tbsp.	60ml
5 Tbsp.	75ml
6 Tbsp.	90ml
7 Tbsp.	105ml

TEMPERATURE CONVERSIONS

CELSIUS	FAHRENHEIT
54.5°C	130°F
60.0°C	140°F
65.5°C	150°F
71.1°C	160°F
76.6°C	170°F
82.2°C	180°F
87.8°C	190°F
93.3°C	200°F
100°C	212°F

Conclusion

Adopting a new way of life can be challenging. It's not so much about the difficulty of the lifestyle as it is about the changes. Every change in your lifestyle is significant, and you must adhere to it. This is where the majority of people fall short.

The way of life we've been leading has become ingrained in our DNA. The trouble you have changing your lifestyle is not due to any technical difficulties but also your habit of doing certain things.

If a healthier life is what you desire, you will need to make this change.
The best part about intermittent fasting is how long it lasts. It's a lifestyle that will easily become a part of your daily routine, making it very long-term. Because there aren't many significant changes to make, the transition is generally not too difficult. However, if you try to make dramatic changes all at once, you will undoubtedly run into difficulties.

Following a 16-hour fasting routine, for example, can be difficult at first if you have never fasted before. This is something you can never do.

Proper Transition Is the Key

When describing the intermittent fasting routine, we already touched on this subject. However, emphasizing its importance is never enough, as it is the single most common cause of failure.

Most women are in such a rush to lose weight and get slim that they want to start with the most challenging routine to get the best results as quickly as possible, and this is where they fail.

You must pay attention to the transition if you want to achieve excellent results and keep them for a long time. The most effective way to begin intermittent fasting is to:

- Start by eliminating snacks
- Practice 12-hour fasts with only three meals in the eating window for as long as you get used to the routine
- Please move to the 14:10 fast and practice it for as long as you get used to it
- You don't have to start following 16:8 fasts as a ritual
- Keep following 14:10 fasts but don't break your fast in the morning until you feel starving
- If you are comfortable, only extend your fasts to 16 hours or longer.

Never extend your fasts longer than 20 hours regularly.

Autophagy is a fantastic process, and you may want to start it as well. It has great health benefits. However, it is difficult, and you should not fast for an extended period without prior preparation. Longer fasts should only be kept after your body has established some knowledge of fasting.

Longer fasts are beneficial, but they should not be done regularly. You should not use them just once every few months. Intermittent fasting regularly can also improve your health.

Recipe Index

www.ingramcontent.com/pod-product-compliance
Lightning Source LLC
Chambersburg PA
CBHW080626030426
42336CB00018B/3099